Healing

An **A-Z guide** to **vitamins**, **minerals** and **supplements**

Supplements

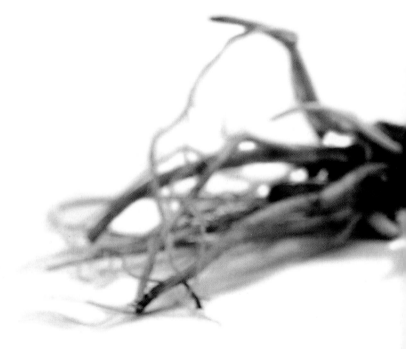

The root of the valerian
plant contains compounds
that promote relaxation
and encourage sleep.

Healing

An **A-Z guide** to **vitamins**, **minerals** and **supplements**

Supplements

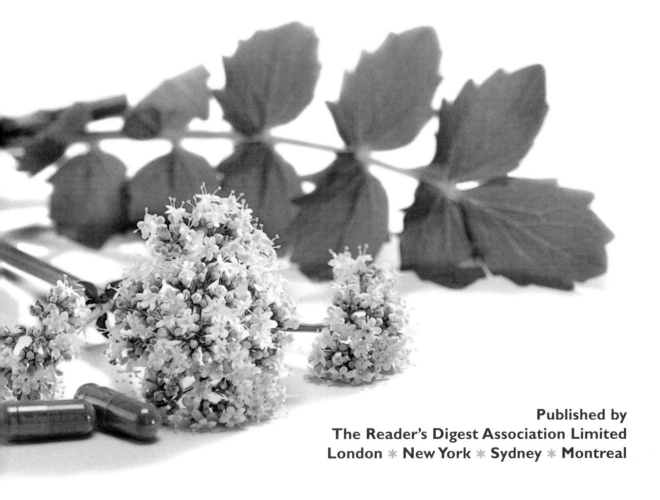

Published by
The Reader's Digest Association Limited
London * **New York** * **Sydney** * **Montreal**

Contents

Introduction

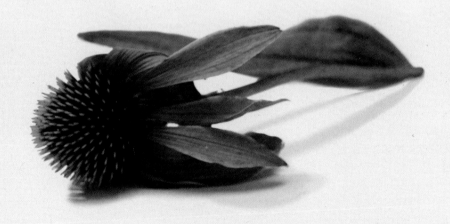

Supplements

These pages are colour-coded: ● vitamins ● minerals ● herbs ● nutritional supplements

The best of health

In the 21st century, our expectation of life is higher than ever thanks to medical advances. With a little care, it could be higher still and our quality of life could be better. The key to lasting good health is good nutrition but many people do not reach their recommended target intakes for vitamins and minerals – perhaps because they fail to take exercise and make poor food choices, missing out on nutrient-rich fruit and vegetables, and wholegrain cereals.

Poor health is often associated with low intakes of essential nutrients. The body's ability to maintain normal healthy functioning of cells depends on 'homeostasis', its self-healing capacity. An important element in this process is the supply of nutrients – each cell requires more than 40 – as well as protective substances, called phytochemicals, from plants.

As many chronic illnesses are the result of years of poor food choice, full health is likely to be restored more quickly if supplements are taken at the same time as the switch to a good diet is made. The inflammation that is associated with asthma, eczema, psoriasis and rheumatoid arthritis, for example, is likely to respond much more quickly to supplementation with vitamins C and E and omega-3 EFAs than to dietary improvement alone – even though achieving improvement through diet is the long-term ideal. You may also find your symptoms disappear more quickly if you take a combination of supplements. This is because all cells require all nutrients at the same time.

The recommendations for the use of the vitamins and minerals described here are based on the results of studies with human subjects; the levels for maximum intakes are based on recommendations from the Expert Group on Vitamins and Minerals (2003). These limits are judged safe for self-administration, although a nutritional therapist might suggest higher levels after a consultation.

Scientific research backs up the historical use of the herbs described in this book; herbs are rich sources of numerous phytochemicals and, like nutrients, they have healing effects on all the body's cells, as well as on specific organs.

Supplements cannot replace a good diet but they can help to make up for nutritional deficiencies resulting from poor lifestyle choices or specific conditions. The wealth of information in this book explores the potential of supplements to boost health and enable many more people to improve their well-being and quality of life.

How supplements can benefit you

A multivitamin and multimineral supplement is often taken as an insurance against nutritional deficiencies, but recent research provides good reasons for using a variety of supplements, including herbs, for both prevention and healing – and indicates that optimum levels may be higher than previously thought.

If you are fundamentally healthy, is there any point in taking supplements on a regular basis? If you develop a disorder or an ailment, can you expect supplements to help? What follows is a summary of the major benefits that, according to scientific researchers, most people can expect if they use the supplements covered in this book. More detailed information about the therapeutic effects of specific supplements can be found in the entries on pages 24-175.

Who needs supplements?

Conventional medical wisdom holds that healthy people who eat well enough to avoid specific nutritional deficiencies do not need to supplement their diets. The only thing they have to do is to make sure that their diets meet the RNIs – Reference Nutrient Intakes – published by the Department of Health (*see page* 10).

Even if you accept that the official standards for vitamin and mineral intakes are adequate for good health, the evidence is overwhelming that most people in the UK fail to come close to meeting those requirements.

Most of us do not eat enough fruit and vegetables, and certainly not as much as five daily servings – the quantity recommended for obtaining the minimum level of nutrients believed necessary to prevent illness.

We often make food choices that are nutritionally poor, selecting chips rather than broccoli as a vegetable serving, for instance, or opting for a fizzy soft drink rather than a glass of semi-skimmed milk. Eating these and other foods may contribute too much fat and sugar to our diet and can also result in intakes of vitamins, minerals and disease-fighting phyto-chemicals that fall well short of ideal levels.

Meeting dietary targets

Government studies show that the diets of many people in the UK contain only half the recommended amounts of magnesium and folic acid. About 50% of adult women and more than 70% of adolescent girls have intakes of calcium that are below their respective RNIs of 700mg and 800mg.

Vitamins C and B_6, as well as iron and zinc, are other nutrients that are at notably low levels in the British diet. Even with the best nutritional planning it is hard to maintain a diet that meets the RNIs for all nutrients. Vegetarians, for example, who as a group are healthier than meat eaters (and who tend to avoid junk foods lacking in vitamins and minerals), may still be deficient in some nutrients, such as iron, calcium and vitamin B_{12}.

People on a low-fat diet will find it difficult to obtain the recommended daily amounts of vitamin E from their food alone, because so many food sources for vitamin E are high in fat. Another problem is that a balanced diet may not contain some of the more specialised substances – fish oils, soya isoflavones or alpha-lipoic acid – that are now believed to promote health.

For a healthy person who is unable to eat a well-balanced diet every day, taking a supplement can fill the nutritional gaps or boost the levels of nutrients they consume from adequate to optimum.

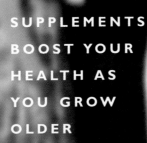

SUPPLEMENTS BOOST YOUR HEALTH AS YOU GROW OLDER

Hazards in the environment

There are various other reasons why people who maintain good eating habits might benefit from a daily supplement. Some practitioners believe that exposure to environmental pollutants – ranging from car emissions to industrial chemicals and wastes – can cause much damage inside the body at the cellular level, destroying tissues and depleting the body of nutrients.

Many supplements, particularly those that act as antioxidants, can help to control the cell and tissue damage that follows toxic exposure (*see* ANTIOXIDANTS, *pages* 30-31). Recent evidence also indicates that certain medications, excessive consumption of alcohol, smoking or persistent stress may interfere with the absorption of certain key nutrients. Even an excellent diet could not make up for such shortfalls. Specific nutritional programmes can be devised that take account of these and other lifestyle factors that affect the nutrient levels in the human body.

Prevention of disease

It used to be thought that a lack of nutrients was linked only to specific deficiency diseases such as scurvy, a condition marked by soft gums and loose teeth that is caused by having too little vitamin C. But in the past three decades thousands of scientific studies have indicated that particular nutrients play important roles in the prevention of a number of chronic degenerative diseases common in contemporary Western societies.

Many recent studies highlighting the disease-fighting potential of different nutrients are mentioned in this book. What most of them reveal is that the level of nutrients associated with the prevention of disease is often much higher than the current RNIs. The people taking part in the studies frequently had to depend on supplements to achieve these higher levels.

Some practitioners suggest that, in slowing or preventing the development of disease, nutrients (particularly the antioxidants) can also delay the wear and tear of ageing itself by reducing the damage done to cells. This does not mean that vitamin E or coenzyme Q_{10}, for example, is a 'youth potion', but several recent studies, including work done at the US Nutritional Immunological Laboratory, have found that supplementation with single nutrients, such as vitamin E, or multivitamin and multimineral supplements seems to improve the immune response in older people.

ANTIOXIDANTS PROVIDE POTENT DEFENCE AGAINST MANY AILMENTS

Age-related disorders

A study of 11,178 elderly subjects by the US National Institute on Aging showed that the use of vitamin E resulted in fewer deaths than would have been expected, especially deaths from heart disease. Vitamin E users were only half as likely to die of heart disease as those who took no supplements. Antioxidant supplements have been shown to be effective in lowering the risk of cataracts and macular degeneration, two age-related conditions in which vision slowly deteriorates. Nutritional supplements that serve as high-potency antioxidants against ageing disorders include selenium, carotenoids, flavonoids, certain amino acids and coenzyme Q_{10}. Research suggests that the herb ginkgo biloba may improve some age-related symptoms, especially those involving reduced blood flow, such as dizziness, impotence and short-term memory loss.

Substances found in echinacea and other herbs are reported to strengthen the immune system, and phytoestrogens such as soya isoflavones may help to delay or prevent some of the effects of the menopause as well as to prevent cancer and heart disease.

Treating ailments

Many practitioners of complementary medicine recommend supplements for a wide range of health problems affecting virtually every system in the body. Traditional doctors would be more likely to prescribe drugs for such conditions, although they might treat some disorders with supplements; for example, iron is sometimes prescribed for some types of anaemia, vitamin A (in the drug isotretinoin) for severe acne, and high doses of the B vitamin niacin for reducing high cholesterol levels.

In this book certain vitamins and minerals are suggested for the treatment of specific ailments – but the use of nutritional supplements as remedies, especially for serious conditions, is controversial. Doctors practising conventional medicine are often sceptical of their efficacy, and believe that it is sometimes dangerous to rely on them. However, drawing on published data and their clinical observations, nutritionally orientated doctors and practitioners think the use of these supplements is justified – and that to wait years for unequivocal proof to appear would be wasting valuable time.

Until there is clearer and more consistent evidence available you should be careful about depending on nutritional supplements alone to treat an ailment or injury.

A tradition of herbal medicine

For thousands of years various cultures have employed herbs for soothing, relieving or even curing many common health problems – a fact not ignored by medical science. After all, the pharmaceutical industry grew out of the tradition of using herbs as medicine.

Recent studies suggest that many of the claims made for herbs are valid, and the pharmacological actions of the herbs covered in this book are often well documented by clinical studies as well as historical practice. A number of herbal remedies, including St John's wort, ginkgo biloba and saw palmetto, are now accepted and prescribed as medications for treating disorders such as allergies, depression, impotence and heart disease. But even herbs and other supplements with proven therapeutic effects should be used judiciously for treating an ailment. Guidelines for using these remedies safely and effectively are given on pages 19-20.

What supplements will not do

Despite the benefits of supplements, it is important to be aware of their limitations – and some of the questionable claims made for them.

■ As the word itself suggests, a 'supplement' is not meant to replace the nutrients available from foods. Supplements can never compensate for a poor diet: they cannot counteract a high intake of saturated fat (linked to an increased risk of heart disease), nor can they replace every nutrient found in food groups that do not form part of your diet. Also, although scientists have isolated and extracted a number of disease-fighting phytochemical compounds from fruit, vegetables and other foods, there may be many others that are undiscovered – and that you can get only from food sources. And some of the known compounds may work only when used in combination with others in various foods, rather than as single ingredients in a supplement form.

■ Supplements cannot compensate for habits that are known to contribute to ill health, such as smoking or lack of exercise. Optimum health requires a wholesome lifestyle – particularly if people, as they get older, are intent on staying active and ageing well.

■ Although some of the benefits ascribed to supplements are unproved but plausible, other claims are far-fetched, particularly those made for some weight-loss preparations. It is questionable whether any such preparation can help you to shed pounds without making the right food choices and taking regular exercise at the same time. Products that claim to 'burn fat' won't burn enough on their own for significant weight loss.

■ Similarly, claims about supplements that are alleged to boost mental or physical performance are difficult to prove – and in a healthy person any 'enhancement' will be at best a limited one. Although a particular supplement may improve mental function in someone experiencing mild to severe episodes of memory loss, it may have a negligible effect on most adults' memories or their ability to concentrate. A supplement that has been shown to counteract fatigue will not transform the average jogger into an endurance athlete. Nor is there any convincing evidence that 'aphrodisiac' supplements are effective in enhancing sexual performance.

■ No supplements are known to have the capacity to cure serious diseases such as cancer, heart disease, diabetes and HIV/AIDS. However, the right supplement may help to improve a chronic condition and to relieve symptoms such as pain and inflammation. But you should always consult your doctor before taking supplements as a treatment for any condition.

THE NUTRIENTS WE NEED

RECOMMENDED DAILY INTAKE OF VITAMINS			
SUPPLEMENT	RNI FOR MALE 19-50	RNI FOR FEMALE 19-50	RDA
Thiamin (mg)	1.0	0.8	1.4
Riboflavin (mg)	1.3	1.1	1.6
Niacin (mg)	17	13	18
Vitamin B$_6$ (mg)	1.4	1.2	2.0
Vitamin B$_{12}$ (mcg)	1.5	1.5	1.0
Folate (mcg)	200	200	200
Vitamin C (mg)	40	40	60
Vitamin A (mcg)	700	600	800
Calcium (mg)	700	700	800
Phosphorus (mg)	550	550	800
Magnesium (mg)	300	270	300
Iron (mg)	8.7	14.8	14
Zinc (mg)	9.5	7	15
Iodine (mcg)	140	140	150
Vitamin E (mg)	no value	no value	10
Selenium (mcg)	75	60	no value
Vitamin D (mcg)	no value	no value	5
Sodium (mg)	1600	1600	no value
Potassium (mcg)	3500	3500	no value
Chloride (mg)	2500	2500	no value
Copper (mg)	1.0	1.2	no value

■ The acronym RNI stands for Reference Nutrient Intake – the amount of a nutrient (as determined by the UK's Department of Health) required daily by the majority of a specified population group, which can differ according to sex and age.

■ RNI values are derived from studies of the physiological requirements of healthy people. For example, the RNI for a vitamin may be based on the amount needed to maintain its correct blood level in a test group of people.

■ RNI values in the UK tend to be modest compared with other countries, especially the USA. An RNI is not the amount of a nutrient recommended for optimum nutrition; despite much research values for optimal intakes are still being debated. Where there is not enough information for an RNI to be set, a Safe Intake (SI) - a level based on maintaining good health, is recommended.

■ RDA – Recommended Daily Amount – is a more general EU approximation, see page 18.

Basic types of supplement

If you visit a health-food shop, or stroll down the dietary supplement aisle in a supermarket or any large pharmacy, you cannot fail to be struck by the huge variety of products on the market.

Taking into account different brands and combinations of supplements, there are literally thousands of choices available. You are not likely to encounter as many as this in one location, but even a far more limited selection in your local chemist's shop can be confusing.

Manufacturers are constantly trying to distinguish their own brands from others, and so they devise different dosages, new combinations and creatively worded claims for their products. At the same time, scientists have found new and better ways of extracting nutritional components from plants and synthesising nutrients in a laboratory, resulting in many new and purer products.

Making informed decisions

In order to find your way through the jungle it is helpful to be familiar with the natures and properties of specific supplements – more than 70 of which are examined in detail in this book. It is also essential to understand the terms used on supplement labels – advice on how to read a label is given on pages 17-18. But, to avoid feeling overwhelmed by all the choices facing you, it is useful first of all to learn about the basic types of supplement that are available and the key functions they perform in helping to keep you healthy.

The characteristics of vitamins, minerals, herbs and other supplements, including phytochemicals, are described below and on the next page. Some substances, such as amino acids, have been known to scientists for many years but only recently marketed as dietary supplements.

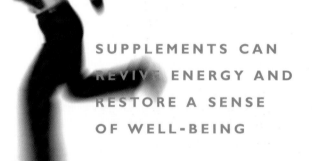

SUPPLEMENTS CAN REVIVE ENERGY AND RESTORE A SENSE OF WELL-BEING

Vitamins

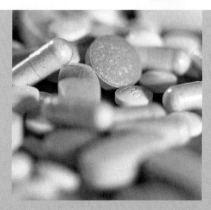

■ A vitamin is an organic substance that is essential for regulating both the metabolic functions within the body's cells and the processes that release energy from food.

■ Evidence is growing that certain vitamins are antioxidants. These are substances that protect tissues from cell damage and may possibly help to prevent a number of degenerative diseases.

■ There are 13 known vitamins, which can be categorised as either fat-soluble (A, D, E and K) or water-soluble (the eight B vitamins and C).

■ The distinction between fat-soluble and water-soluble vitamins is important because the body stores fat-soluble vitamins for relatively long periods, such as months or even years; on the other hand, water-soluble vitamins, except vitamin B_{12}, remain in the body for a short time and therefore need to be replenished more frequently.

■ With a few exceptions, notably vitamins D and K, the body does not have the capacity to manufacture vitamins – so, to maintain good health, they must be ingested through food or in nutritional supplements.

Minerals

- Minerals are present in the body in small amounts: in total they add up to only 4% of body weight.
- These inorganic substances are essential for a wide range of vital processes, from basic bone formation to the normal functioning of the heart and digestive system.
- A number of minerals have been linked to the prevention of cancer, osteoporosis and other chronic illnesses.
- Humans must replenish their mineral supplies through food or with supplements.
- Of more than 60 different minerals in the body, only 22 are considered essential.
- Of these, seven – including calcium, chloride, magnesium, phosphorus, potassium, sodium and sulphur – are usually called macrominerals, or major minerals.
- The other 15 minerals are called trace minerals, or microminerals, because the amount needed each day for good health is tiny (usually measured in micrograms, or millionths of a gram).

Herbs

- Herbal supplements are prepared from plants, often using the leaves, stems, roots and/or bark, as well as the buds and flowers.
- Many plant parts can be either used in their natural forms, or refined into tablets, capsules, powders, tinctures and other formulations.
- A herbal supplement may contain all the compounds found in a plant, or just one or two of the isolated compounds that have been successfully extracted.
- Many herbs have several active compounds that interact with one another to produce a therapeutic effect.
- In some herbs the active agents simply have not been identified, so it is necessary to use the entire herb to obtain all its benefits.
- Of the hundreds of remedies that feature in the current rebirth of interest in herbal medicines, the majority are used to treat chronic or mild health problems.
- Herbs are also used to attain or maintain good health – for example, to enhance the immune system, to help to keep cholesterol levels low or to protect against fatigue.

Other supplements

- These nutrients include a diverse group of products. Some, such as fish oils, are food substances believed by scientists to possess disease-fighting potential.
- Flavonoids, soya isoflavones, and carotenoids are phyto-chemicals – compounds found in fruit and vegetables that work to lower the risk of disease and may alleviate the symptoms of some ailments.
- Other nutritional supplements, such as coenzyme Q_{10}, are substances present in the body that can be re-created synthetically in a laboratory.
- Among similar examples is acidophilus, a 'friendly' bacterium in the body that, taken as a supplement, may aid in the treatment of some digestive disorders.
- Amino acids are the building blocks for proteins that may play a role in strengthening the immune system and in other health-promoting activities and are now available as supplements.

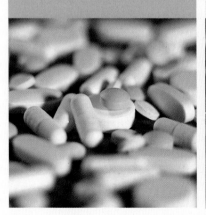

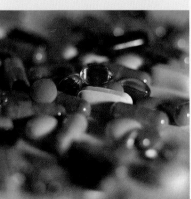

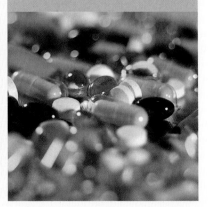

Buying supplements: preparations and forms

The number of different forms and strengths of supplements available theoretically allows you to find the kind that is best for you, but the wide choice and the varying label claims can make shopping for supplements confusing.

Some 'special' formulas – including those described as 'timed-release' or 'chelated' – may provide little additional benefit and are often not worth the extra expense.

Common forms

Tablets and capsules are frequently the most convenient forms of supplement to use, but other forms may be more appropriate in some cases.

TABLETS AND CAPSULES

Both tablets and capsules are easy to use and store, and they generally have a longer life than some other supplement forms. As well as their vitamin or nutrient content, tablets are also likely to contain more, usually inert, additives known as excipients. These compounds bind, preserve or give bulk to the supplement, and some can help tablets to break down more quickly in the stomach. Increasingly, supplements are available in capsule-shaped, easy-to-swallow 'caplets'.

Essential fatty acids, such as those found in fish oils and evening primrose oil, and sometimes the fat-soluble vitamins A, D and E are available as 'softgel' capsules. Other vitamins and minerals are processed into powders or liquids and then encapsulated.

Capsules tend to have fewer additives than tablets, and there is evidence that they dissolve more readily, although this does not necessarily mean that they are absorbed better by the body.

POWDERS

People who find pills hard to swallow may choose to use powders, which can be mixed into juice or water or stirred into food. Ground seeds such as psyllium often come in this form.

ABOUT THE LABEL CLAIMS

- Advertising claims imply that vitamins derived from 'natural' sources – vitamin E from soya beans, for example – are better than 'synthetic' vitamins created chemically in a laboratory.
- Makers may state that their products are 'natural' but most supplements, no matter what their source, will have undergone some kind of processing.
- The term 'natural' on a label highlights the fact that nutrients have been extracted from a food or another natural source – but they may have been greatly altered from their original states.
- Even synthetic vitamins derived from a natural starting material may be described as 'natural' – such as vitamin C made from corn syrup. 'Natural extracts', on the other hand, are simply extracts of concentrated food formulated to produce a higher nutrient content.
- Some manufacturers describe their synthetic nutrients as 'nature identical' because, whether a nutrient is synthetic or natural, the chemical structure is identical, and the human body is unable to distinguish between the two.
- Manufacturers can make synthetic products more concentrated, producing smaller-sized supplements that are easier to swallow. Synthetic products are not as sensitive as non-synthetic versions to the effects of heat and light.
- If additives, fillers and binders – also known as excipients, or non-active ingredients – are added to a supplement, the person who takes the supplement actually receives less of the active ingredients. This means that in order to obtain the required dosage of the nutrient, more supplements have to be taken.
- Before using a supplement, always check the ingredients list; this is particularly important if you suffer from any allergic reactions.

Powdered vitamin C can be mixed with water for use as a skin compress. Dosages of powders can be easily adjusted, and because single nutrient powders have fewer additives than tablets or capsules they are useful for individuals who are allergic to certain substances. Powders are often cheaper than tablets or capsules.

LIQUIDS

Liquid formulas for oral use are easy to swallow and can be flavoured; many children's formulas are in liquid form. Some supplements, such as vitamin E, also come in this form for applying topically to the skin.

CHEWABLE TABLETS

Such supplements are usually flavoured, and are particularly useful for people who have trouble swallowing pills. They do not need to be taken with water.

Deglycyrrhised liquorice (DGL) is activated by saliva, so the tablets should be chewed rather than simply swallowed. Vitamin C is often found in chewable form. These tablets are often high in sugar or artificial sweeteners.

LOZENGES

Some supplements can be bought in the form of lozenges that dissolve slowly in the mouth. Zinc lozenges, for example, help in the treatment of colds and flu.

SUBLINGUAL LIQUIDS AND TABLETS

A few supplements in liquid or tablet form are formulated to dissolve sublingually (under the tongue), providing quick absorption into the bloodstream without interference from stomach acids and digestive enzymes.

TIMED-RELEASE FORMULAS

These consist of tiny capsules contained within a standard-size capsule. The microcapsules gradually break down, releasing the vitamin into the bloodstream over a period of about 2 to 10 hours. Vitamin C is often sold in this form because it cannot be stored in the body. Timed-release formulas may allow a more natural and even absorption of a vitamin into the blood-stream, but there are no reliable studies showing that they are more efficiently utilised by the body than conventional capsules or tablets.

CHELATED MINERALS

Minerals in supplements are chelated, or bonded, to another substance; this may be an inorganic mineral, an organic substance or an amino acid. The substance to which a mineral is chelated dictates how well it is absorbed. Inorganic chelates, such as oxides, sulphates, phosphates, chlorides and carbonates, tend to be cheaper than organic chelates but less well absorbed. Organic chelates, including ascorbates, citrates, succinates and malates, are better absorbed.

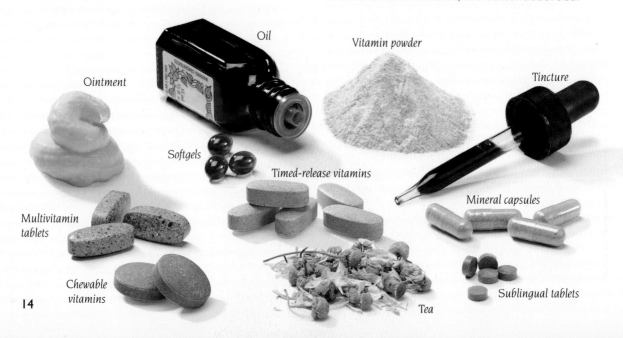

Oil

Vitamin powder

Tincture

Ointment

Softgels

Timed-release vitamins

Mineral capsules

Multivitamin tablets

Chewable vitamins

Tea

Sublingual tablets

Herbal remedies

You can buy whole herbs and make up your own formulas, but the tablets, capsules and other prepackaged forms described below, including forms for external use, are readily available in supermarkets, chemists' and health-food shops.

There are also many different preparations that combine one herb with another, or combine herbs with other nutritional supplements.

TABLETS AND CAPSULES

Tablets and capsules are prepared using either a whole herb or an extract containing a high concentration of the herb's active components. Either form allows you to avoid the often bitter taste of the herb. The constituents are ground into a powder that can be pressed into tablets or encapsulated.

Some herbs are available in 'enteric'-coated capsules. These pass through the stomach into the small intestine before dissolving. This minimises potential gastrointestinal discomfort and also enhances the absorption of some herbs into the bloodstream.

TINCTURES

These concentrated liquids are made by soaking the whole or part of a herb in water and alcohol. The alcohol acts to extract and concentrate the herb's active components. In certain cases some or all of the alcohol is then removed. Non-alcoholic concentrations can also be made using glycerine.

Tinctures are typically taken in small doses several times a day. The dose is measured in drops with a pipette and usually diluted in water or juice.

TEAS, INFUSIONS AND DECOCTIONS

Less concentrated than tinctures, teas and infusions are brewed from the fresh or dried flowers, leaves or roots of a herb. They can be purchased in bulk or as tea

bags. Although tea is normally made with boiling water, the herbal teas recommended in this book are prepared as infusions, using hot water that is just on the verge of boiling – this preserves the beneficial oils that can be dissipated by the steam of boiling water. To make a decoction the tougher parts of a herb, such as the stem or bark, are generally simmered for at least half an hour.

These liquid remedies should be used as soon as possible after being brewed because they start to lose their potency within a few hours of exposure to air. If stored in tightly sealed glass jars in the refrigerator they will retain some strength for up to three days.

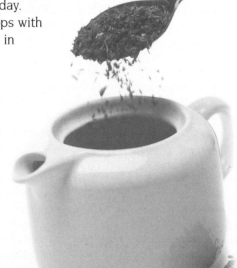

ESSENTIAL OILS

Oils extracted from herbs can be distilled to form potent concentrations for external use in massage or on particular areas of the skin. These 'essential' oils are usually placed in a neutral 'carrier' oil, such as almond oil, before use on the skin. (Milder 'infused' oils can be prepared at home.) Essential herbal oils should never be ingested, with one exception – a few drops of peppermint oil on the tongue may be recommended for bad breath, and capsules of the same oil can be beneficial in the treatment of digestive problems.

GELS, OINTMENTS AND CREAMS

Gels and ointments made from the fats or oils of aromatic herbs are applied to the skin to soothe rashes, heal bruises or wounds and serve other therapeutic purposes. Creams are usually light oil-and-water mixtures that are partly absorbed by the skin, allowing it to breathe while also keeping in moisture. Creams can be used for moisturising dry skin, for cleansing, and for relieving rashes, insect bites or sunburn.

Standardised extracts

To obtain a concentrated extract, a herb is soaked in alcohol or water (which is allowed to evaporate) and then put into a heavy press. Extracts are the most effective form of herbs, which makes them particularly useful for people with absorption difficulties or severe disorders.

When herbs are recommended in this book for the treatment of ailments, it is usually suggested that 'standardised extracts' should be chosen. Herbalists and manufacturers use this term to guarantee the potency of the active ingredients of a product.

The quality of a herb is dependent on many factors, including the sunlight, temperature, soil quality and water to which it was exposed when growing as well as storage conditions and extraction and manufacturing procedures. A change in any of these conditions can affect potency. The standardisation of an extract ensures that the product you are buying is not affected by these variations.

To achieve standardisation the active components of a whole herb – such as the allicin in garlic or the ginsenosides in ginseng – are extracted, concentrated and made into a form of supplement, such as a

THE 'HYPE' FACTOR

To distinguish one brand from another, supplement manufacturers have developed their own jargon in promoting their products. The following terms commonly appear on supplement labels and in advertisements. Each term implies a superior product, but none has a standard definition agreed upon by experts or by the regulations governing the manufacture and sale of supplements. Pay attention to the specific ingredients and directions on a label rather than the 'hype' of these terms:

- Clinically proven
- Highly concentrated
- Maximum absorption
- Natural (or naturally occurring)
- Nutritionally comprehensive
- Pure
- Quality extract
- Scientifically standardised

tablet, capsule or tincture. By this method a precise amount of the active ingredient can be supplied in each dose.

Sometimes, instead of standardised extracts, manufacturers process the whole, or crude, herb. In this case the whole herb is simply air or freeze-dried, made into a powder then converted into capsule, tablet, tincture or other form ready for packaging.

Herbalists continue to debate the comparative merits of standardised extracts and crude herbs. Crude herbs may contain unidentified active ingredients, and only by ingesting the whole thing can all its benefits be obtained. In many cases you would have to use a much greater amount of a whole herb to gain an effect similar to that of a standardised product, but although standardised products are more consistent from batch to batch, this does not mean that they are more effective.

Buying supplements: how to read a label

Understanding the key terms that may be found on supplement labels can help you to make a better informed decision about which supplement is right for you.

Manufacturers are required by law not to be misleading about their products. However, because there is no standardisation of information with regard to supplements, you are likely to see differences in the wording and details that appear on packaging.

Health-improving claims

Most nutritional supplements for sale in the UK are classed as foods, which restricts what can be said about them. A limited number of health maintenance claims are allowed, but suggesting that such a product has the property to treat, prevent or cure any condition is prohibited.

Certain products with a licence granted by the Medicines and Healthcare Products Regulatory Agency (MHRA) can cite health-improving claims. This is why you may read on an echinacea bottle 'a traditional herbal remedy for the symptomatic relief of colds and influenza', but packaging for vitamin C could usually only go as far as to say that the product is 'important for a healthy immune system'. If a vitamin C product is licensed for the relief of colds, however, then the label could make that claim. There are licensed vitamin supplements on the market – look for a PL (Product Licence) number on the packaging.

What the terms mean

QUANTITY The amount in the container, in terms either of the number of capsules or tablets or volume or weight.

'HIGH POTENCY' This term could be used to compare the strengths of different products in a manufacturer's range, but it can be misleading without other information. It is better to check nutrient quantities and compare them with other products than to set store by this term.

DIRECTIONS FOR USE Instructions on the amount of the supplement to take, as recommended by the manufacturer. This normally includes advice about when and how to take the product – with or between meals or with a glass of water, for

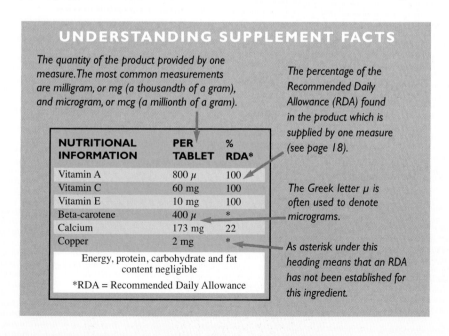

UNDERSTANDING SUPPLEMENT FACTS

The quantity of the product provided by one measure. The most common measurements are milligram, or mg (a thousandth of a gram), and microgram, or mcg (a millionth of a gram).

The percentage of the Recommended Daily Allowance (RDA) found in the product which is supplied by one measure (see page 18).

NUTRITIONAL INFORMATION	PER TABLET	% RDA*
Vitamin A	800 μ	100
Vitamin C	60 mg	100
Vitamin E	10 mg	100
Beta-carotene	400 μ	*
Calcium	173 mg	22
Copper	2 mg	*
Energy, protein, carbohydrate and fat content negligible		
*RDA = Recommended Daily Allowance		

The Greek letter μ is often used to denote micrograms.

As asterisk under this heading means that an RDA has not been established for this ingredient.

example. If a product is classed as a food it should not refer to a 'dose' or 'dosage', which suggests a medical use.

INGREDIENTS A list of everything in the supplement, arranged in decreasing order according to weight, is required by law. Ingredients include binders, fillers, coatings, preservatives, colouring agents and other substances, including inert ones.

CAUTION A statement warning that, for example, pregnant women or those with an allergy to niacin should not use a product, or to advise that a doctor should be consulted if a user is under medical supervision. Cautions about the dangers of exceeding the stated measure of vitamin A and iron are required by law.

CHILD WARNING A precautionary statement that all supplements should be kept in a place where children cannot reach them. Some supplements can be toxic to children in large amounts.

STORAGE ADVICE This is advice on how best to store the product. When this information appears on a bottle or packet it is found next to the 'best before' date or a reference to it. Most supplements should be kept in a cool, dry place, which means they should not be stored in a refrigerator or in a damp place where moisture could cause damage to them. There are, however, some products that should be refrigerated after opening. If this is the case, the label on the product will tell you.

'BEST BEFORE' DATE A date up to which the supplement can be expected to retain its full potency, if properly stored. In effect, it is a pledge from the manufacturer that the product will remain 'fresh' up to that point.

NAME AND PLACE OF BUSINESS The name and address of the manufacturer, packager or distributor. This is the address you can write to for more product information. There may also be a telephone number on the label.

UNDERSTANDING 'BP'
■ You may see the letters 'BP' on the packaging of some supplements. This is the stamp of the British Pharmacopoeia, a commission that is appointed by the government and works closely with the Medicines and Healthcare products Regulatory Agency (MHRA).
■ A BP specification for a particular preparation, sometimes known as a monograph, provides an indication that the product contains the right amount of the right active ingredient of the right quality.
■ 'BP' on the label indicates that the quality of the ingredients has been checked, even though their potency has not necessarily been assessed. For products that are intended for medicinal use it applies whether or not the letters 'BP' appear on the label.
■ Products that are not sold for medicinal purposes, such as certain vitamins, do not have to comply with the BP, but are permitted to carry the designation if they are of the required quality.

WHY DO LABELS USE THE TERM RDA?

■ As required by European Union regulations, labels on foods and dietary supplements give their contents of nutrients as Recommended Daily Amounts (RDAs).
■ RDAs approximate to the average quantities of key nutrients that 'average adults' should obtain from their diets.
■ Since they are based on very general requirements, RDAs are only a very rough guide to healthy eating – they take no account of differences in individual nutritional requirements according to age, gender or other factors. For example, an RDA does not differentiate between a man of 18 and a woman of 45, who have very different dietary needs.
■ The EU RDA is therefore a simple approximation that is used for labels only.
■ For all other purposes, including the provision of nutritional advice, the UK's Dietary Reference Values (DRVs), including Reference Nutrient Intakes (RNIs, see page 10) are used.

Using supplements safely and effectively

Responsible manufacturers print instructions about proper use on their supplement labels, but you may encounter many brands that do not include instructions.

The entries in this book provide detailed information about the benefits, uses, side effects and forms of supplements, as well as the doses that are considered safe and effective. Below are some general guidelines about the safe and effective use of supplements, and on pages 176-179 you will find a section listing interactions between supplements and commonly prescribed medications.

The proper balance

Some nutrients may interact with one another, which can affect their absorption or utilisation by the body. For example, fat-soluble vitamins (A, D, E and K) require some dietary fat to facilitate absorption so they should be taken with food.

Iron taken with meals is best absorbed with small amounts of meat and foods containing vitamin C. Calcium absorption is improved by taking supplements with meals, and the effect of calcium on building healthy bones is enhanced when it is taken with magnesium.

Other nutrients, when taken in combination, likewise enhance one another's benefits. For example, vitamin C helps to regenerate vitamin E after it has been modified by neutralising reactive free radicals – so, because these antioxidant nutrients work together, they are best taken at the same time.

The proper amounts

Dietary supplements are generally safe when consumed in the appropriate dosages. But more is not necessarily better – and sometimes it can be worse. For example, the mineral selenium is recommended for many disorders, from cataracts to cancer prevention, but taking doses even slightly higher than those recommended can cause loss of hair and other toxic reactions. When using supplements it is advisable to avoid high doses, particularly the extremely high ones known as 'megadoses'.

Whatever the circumstances, follow dosage recommendations closely. In addition, notify your doctor at once if your condition worsens or if any serious adverse reactions develop.

VITAMINS AND MINERALS

Most vitamins can be taken in significantly higher doses than their RNIs (*see page* 10) without incurring adverse reactions. However, some fat-soluble vitamins, which are stored in the body rather than excreted, may be toxic at high doses. In particular, taking an excessive amount of vitamin A or vitamin D is dangerous. Although very high doses of some other vitamins – such as vitamin C – are not toxic, certain individuals may experience side effects. Reducing the dosage will usually remedy the situation.

Some minerals taken in large doses or over time can block the absorption of other minerals; zinc, for instance, can impede the absorption of copper. Also, large amounts of certain minerals are linked to disease – several studies have shown that too much iron in men, for example, increases their risk of heart disease. For these reasons, even researchers who believe that the RNIs for many vitamins are too low think that the levels for minerals are generally adequate for optimum health.

HERBS

Surveys by toxicologists conclude that serious side effects or toxic reactions associated with herbal medicines are rare; nevertheless, some once-popular medicinal herbs, such as foxglove and chaparral, are now recognised as toxic.

Occasionally some people have serious allergic reactions to a herb; these may include a rash or difficulty in breathing. Furthermore, because no uniform quality control for herbal preparations exists, the chemical composition of a herbal remedy can vary greatly from batch to batch. It may also contain potentially toxic contaminants and other ingredients that could influence the herb's effectiveness or cause side effects.

Products that contain standardised extracts are more likely to provide a proper dose of a particular supplement than those that do not, but whenever you buy a supplement – whether it is a standardised extract or a whole herb in tablet, tincture or another form – you are always dependent on the manufacturer's integrity.

PEOPLE WHO SHOULD BE WARY OF HERBS

Using some herbs for medicinal purposes can be dangerous for people with certain conditions or for those on particular medications (*see pages* 176-179). Garlic, for example, may intensify the effects of anticoagulant drugs, while liquorice – which aids digestive problems and enhances the immune system – can raise blood pressure. Even so, apart from the few contraindications that have been identified, the tonic herbs described in this book have no adverse effects and can be safely taken over the long term.

The issue of quality control

How do you know what a product contains? Manufacturers are required by law to list all the active ingredients on each label, but monitoring of the contents of supplements can be sporadic, so no one is sure about the degree of compliance.

Established manufacturers of supplements have reputations to protect, and so they try to ensure that their products contain what is stated on the labels. But herbal supplements can sometimes be problematic.

For example, in a survey sponsored by the Good Housekeeping Institute of America, the levels of an active ingredient in St John's wort were found to vary considerably between brands. A study published in the leading British medical journal *The Lancet* reported that some supplements that purported to be ginseng contained varying amounts of active ginsenosides, and others none at all. However, it was later pointed out that the latter (although called 'ginseng') were actually different species and could not be expected to contain ginsenosides.

SAFETY GUIDELINES

Supplements, especially herbs, can have potent primary effects and side effects, so keep these points in mind when using them:

■ Shop carefully. There is no independent guarantee of purity or potency, so it is up to you to select brands with a reputation for quality.

■ Do not exceed the recommended dosages. Overdosing with a supplement can have serious consequences. In the case of herbs and nutritional supplements, start with the lowest dose when a dosage range is given.

■ Monitor your reactions. At the first sign of a problem, stop using the supplement. You should also stop taking the herb if it does not seem to be working (but give it time – you may need to take a herb for a month or more before noticing an effect).

■ Take a break. If you are treating a particular condition with supplements, it is advisable to take them for specified periods, then stop temporarily to see if the condition has improved. If the problem returns you may need to take the supplement over a long period as a 'maintenance' medication.

■ Avoid risks. If you have symptoms that indicate a serious problem, do not self-treat it with supplements but arrange to see your doctor immediately.

■ Very young or elderly people and pregnant or breastfeeding women, should also consult their doctors before using supplements.

■ Always ask your doctor or pharmacist about possible interactions with any drugs you are taking (see *pages* 176-179).

Practitioners

If you are suffering from a particular ailment, consult your GP for at least an initial diagnosis. In general, practitioners of complementary medicine have less training in making diagnoses, and most would recommend that you see a conventionally trained doctor, particularly for more serious ailments. The two approaches can usually work alongside each other. Your GP may be able to recommend an alternative practitioner, or friends and family may be able to make personal recommendations.

Because anyone can legally call themselves a herbalist, even after completing a course as short as a week, you should obtain a register of accredited practitioners in your area. The Complementary Medical Association and the Institute for Complementary Medicine can provide details of registered naturopaths, herbalists and nutritionists as well as other complementary medicine practitioners (*see pages 180-181*). Registered practitioners have usually completed an accredited course, are insured and have accepted their organisation's code of ethics.

Practitioners should be willing to talk to you on the telephone, explaining their approach and answering your questions. Be wary of anyone who suggests a long, and probably expensive, course of treatment, and of any practitioner who is very dismissive of other approaches. During the initial consultation you should be asked for a full medical history and also for details of any drugs or supplements you are taking – to ensure that any possible adverse interaction between them is avoided. The number and frequency of follow-up visits will depend on the ailment and the practitioner.

MEDICAL HERBALISTS

Although medical herbalists learn the same diagnostic skills as ordinary doctors, they take a holistic approach to healing and use herbs rather than drugs. A member of the National Institute of Medical Herbalists has had four years of training.

NATUROPATHS

Naturopaths are trained in diagnostic skills. Their approach is based on principles which involve non-suppression of symptoms and non-interference with the body's natural defence systems. Treatment may include nutritional advice, hydrotherapy and relaxation techniques.

The letters ND after a name mean that a naturopath has acquired a national diploma after a four-year degree course. The letters MRN indicate a practitioner who is a member of the General Council and Register of Naturopaths, the largest in the UK, which recognises only full-time degree courses.

NUTRITIONISTS

These practitioners specialise in the study of nutrition. The letters RNUT denote a registered nutritionist, while RPHNUT indicates a registered public health nutritionist who has studied 'population' nutrition – for example, in regard to elderly people or some other population group. To be registered with the Nutrition Society a nutritionist must complete a three-year degree course and three years' practical experience.

PHARMACISTS

These are often the most accessible kind of health professional. Although their role is to manage and check the safety and accuracy of prescription drugs, they can also advise patients on how to manage their medicines for optimum treatment. This usually means conventional medicine, but some pharmacists are also knowledgeable about supplements. Any trained pharmacist has completed a four-year degree course and should be registered with the Royal Pharmaceutical Society of Great Britain.

Using this book

In this book you will find detailed profiles of more than 70 popular supplements, arranged alphabetically from aloe vera to zinc. Each entry is colour-coded according to basic supplement type (for a general explanation of these basic types see pages 11-12).

Look for:

- ○ Vitamins
- ● Minerals
- ● Herbs
- ● Nutritional Supplements

Each profile describes what the supplement is, the forms in which it comes and the way it works to promote good health and to prevent or relieve specific ailments. How much you need, the amount you should take at any one time and other guidelines for using the supplement are explained, along with possible side effects. Key food sources of vitamins and minerals are also indicated.

The book also includes special features on antioxidants, functional and fortified foods, and phytochemicals.

However, if you have any serious medical or psychiatric condition — or one that may not have been properly diagnosed — always consult your doctor before treating it with any supplement.

ABOUT THE RECOMMENDATIONS

Specific dosage suggestions are listed in each of the profiles that follow. These are the total daily amount of a supplement that you need to treat a disorder or condition. In practical terms you may have to adjust these numbers to take account of the additional amounts of these same nutrients that you may be getting in any daily multivitamin or individual supplements that you are taking for other health reasons.

For example, we suggest taking 250 mg vitamin E daily for the promotion of a healthy prostate gland. If you are already taking a daily multivitamin tablet that supplies 250 mg vitamin E, you do not need any additional supplement of that vitamin. If you also have angina (which calls for 500 mg vitamin E),

you will have to take only 250 mg more each day to meet that requirement as well. The dosages are meant to be accurate, but each person is different. Always read the label on a supplement packet, and do not exceed recommended dosages, even though you may be treating several ailments. If you have a serious medical condition, consult your doctor about using supplements.

A final word: We have tried to include widely available dosages in the pages that follow but the strengths of individual supplement products vary greatly. If the information on a bottle or packet confuses you, there are many qualified people, including health professionals and pharmicists, who can help you to choose the appropriate dose.

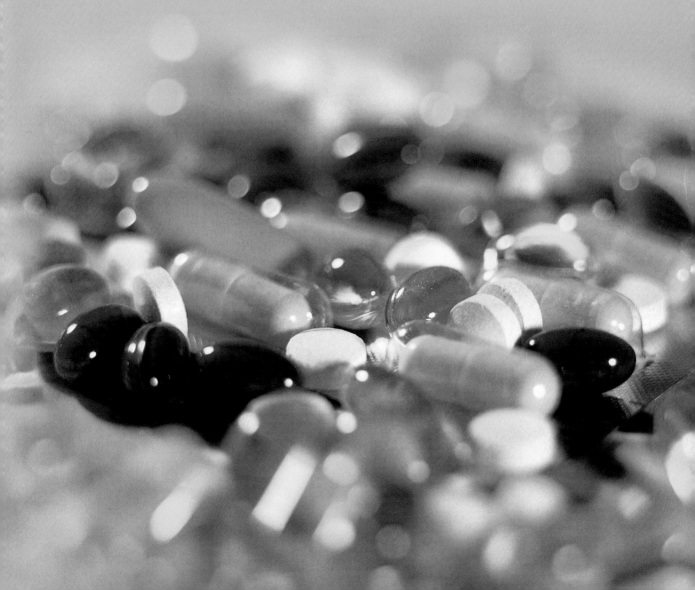

Aloe vera

Aloe vera
A. barbadensis
A. vulgaris

Long before the reign of Cleopatra, the ancient Egyptians discovered the power of the aloe vera plant. The cool, soothing gel from its leaf has been used ever since to treat burns and minor wounds, and is the basis of aloe vera juice, which is effective in calming digestive complaints.

Common uses

Applied topically

- *Heals minor burns (including sunburn), cuts and abrasions, insect bites and stings, small skin ulcers and frostbite.*

- *Relieves the itching of shingles (herpes zoster).*

- *May help to clear up warts.*

Taken internally

- *Soothes ulcers, indigestion and other digestive complaints.*

Forms

- Capsule
- Cream/ointment
- Fresh herb/gel
- Liquid
- Softgel

What it is

A succulent of the lily family, aloe vera has fleshy leaves that provide a gel widely used as a topical treatment for skin problems – a practice dating back to at least 1500 BC, when Egyptian healers described it in their treatises. The plant is native to the Cape of Good Hope and grows wild in much of Africa and Madagascar. Commercial growers cultivate it in the Caribbean, the Mediterranean, Japan and the USA.

What it does

Scientists are not sure how aloe vera works, but they have identified many of its active ingredients. Rich in anti-inflammatory substances, the gel contains a gummy material called acemannan that acts as an emollient, as well as bradykininase, a compound that reduces pain and swelling, and components which sooth itching. Aloe vera also dilates the tiny blood vessels known as capillaries, allowing more blood to reach the site of an injury and thereby speeding up the process of healing. Some studies show that it destroys, or at least inhibits the spread of, a number of bacteria, viruses and fungi.

CAUTION!

- Aloe vera should not be confused with the bitter yellow aloe latex, a laxative which can cause severe cramps and diarrhoea. Pregnant or breast-feeding women, in particular, should avoid aloe latex.

REMINDER: If you have a medical condition, consult your doctor before taking supplements.

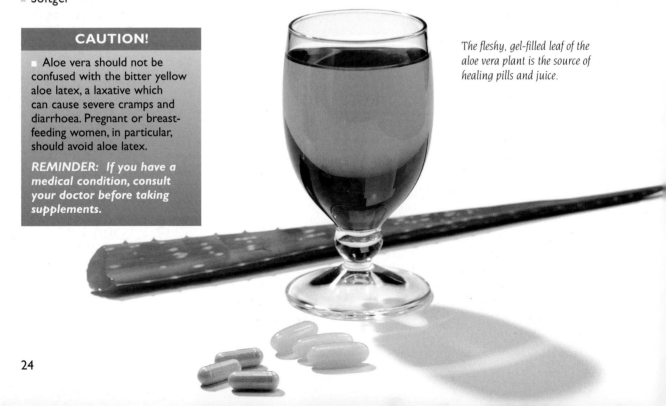

The fleshy, gel-filled leaf of the aloe vera plant is the source of healing pills and juice.

MAJOR BENEFITS: Aloe vera gel is particularly effective when applied to damaged skin. It aids in the healing of minor burns, sunburn, mouth ulcers and minor skin wounds, as well as relieving pain and reducing itching in people suffering from shingles. The gel also provides a hygienic moisturising barrier, so that wounds do not dry out. Its capillary-dilating properties increase blood circulation, speeding the regeneration of skin and alleviating mild cases of frostbite. The gel's antiviral effects may also promote the healing of warts.

Though effective against minor cuts and abrasions, aloe vera may not be a good choice for more serious, infected wounds. In a study of 21 women in a Los Angeles hospital whose caesarean-section wounds had become infected, applying aloe vera gel actually increased the length of time it took for the wounds to heal – from 53 to 83 days.

ADDITIONAL BENEFITS: Aloe vera gel is used to make a juice that may be taken internally to combat inflammatory digestive disorders, including ulcers and indigestion. However, research into its effectiveness in this form has been very limited. In Japan, purified aloe vera compounds have been found to inhibit stomach secretions and lesions. In one study, aloe vera juice cured 17 out of 18 patients with peptic ulcers, but there was no comparison group taking a placebo. A commercial laboratory in the USA is conducting trials with an aloe-derived compound as a treatment for people with ulcerative colitis, a common type of inflammatory bowel disease.

Other studies are exploring aloe vera's effectiveness as a possible antiviral and immune-boosting agent for people suffering from AIDS; as a treatment for victims of leukaemia and other types of cancer; and as a therapy for diabetics.

How to take it

DOSAGE: *For external use*: Liberally apply aloe vera gel or cream to the injured skin as needed or desired. *For internal use*: Take a half to three-quarters of a cup of aloe vera juice three times a day; or take one or two capsules as directed on the label.

GUIDELINES FOR USE: Topically, aloe vera gel can be applied repeatedly, especially in the case of burns. Simply rub it on the affected area, let it dry and reapply when needed. Fresh gel from a live leaf is the most potent – and economical – form of the herb. If you have an aloe vera plant, cut off several inches from a leaf, then slice the cutting lengthwise. Spread the gel found in the centre onto the affected area. For internal use, take aloe vera juice between meals. Aloe latex, a yellow extract from the inner leaf of the plant, is a powerful laxative that should be used only sparingly on the advice of a doctor.

Possible side effects

Topical aloe vera is very safe. On rare occasions a mild itching or rash may develop; if this happens to you, simply discontinue use. Aloe vera juice may – as the result of poor processing – contain small amounts of the laxative ingredient found in aloe latex. If you experience cramping, diarrhoea or loose stools after taking the juice, stop taking it immediately and replace it with a new supply. Never take aloe vera juice if you are pregnant or breastfeeding.

Alpha-lipoic acid

Supplements of alpha-lipoic acid have been shown to alleviate the effects of nerve damage in people with diabetes. They may also protect the liver and brain cells, prevent cataracts and serve as a powerful general antioxidant.

Common uses

- Relieves numbness, tingling and other symptoms of nerve damage in people with diabetes.
- Protects the liver in hepatitis sufferers, and in cases of alcohol abuse, or exposure to poisons or toxic chemicals.
- Inhibits the development of cataracts.
- May help to preserve memory in people with Alzheimer's disease.
- Acts as a high-potency antioxidant and, possibly, an immunity booster; may alleviate a wide range of disorders, including psoriasis, chronic fatigue syndrome and AIDS.

Forms

- Capsule
- Tablet

CAUTION!

■ People suffering from diabetes should take alpha-lipoic acid supplements only under a doctor's supervision.

REMINDER: If you have a medical condition, consult your doctor before taking supplements.

What it is

It had been known since the 1950s that alpha-lipoic acid (also called thioctic acid or, simply, lipoic acid) worked with enzymes throughout the body to speed up the processes involved in energy production. More recently, in the late 1980s, it was discovered that this vitamin-like substance also had the capacity to act as a powerful antioxidant, neutralising naturally occurring, highly reactive molecules called free radicals that can damage cells. Although the body manufactures alpha-lipoic acid in minute amounts, it is mainly present in foods such as spinach, meats (especially liver) and brewer's yeast. It is difficult to obtain therapeutic amounts of alpha-lipoic acid through diet alone, however, and some people find that they need to take supplements in order to benefit fully from its healing properties.

What it does

Alpha-lipoic acid affects nearly every cell in the body. It helps all the B vitamins – including thiamin, riboflavin, pantothenic acid and niacin – to convert carbohydrates, protein and fats found in foods into energy that the body can store for later use. Alpha-lipoic acid is a cell-protecting antioxidant that may stimulate the body to recycle other antioxidants, such as vitamins C and E, thereby boosting their potency. Owing to its unique chemical properties, alpha-lipoic acid is easily absorbed by most tissues in the body, including the brain, nerves and liver, which makes it valuable for treating a wide range of ailments.

✪ **MAJOR BENEFITS:** One of alpha-lipoic acid's primary uses is to treat nerve damage, including the effects of diabetic neuropathy, a long-term complication of diabetes that causes pain and loss of feeling in the limbs. The nervous condition may be partly the result of free-radical damage to nerve cells caused by runaway levels of glucose in the blood. Alpha-lipoic acid may play a role in countering nerve damage through its antioxidant action. In addition, it can help people with diabetes to respond to insulin,

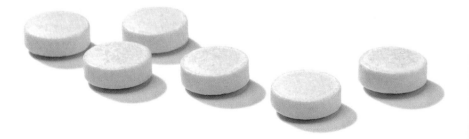

the hormone that regulates glucose levels. In a study of 74 people with type II diabetes who were given 600 mg or more of alpha-lipoic acid daily, all benefited from lowered glucose levels. Studies in animals also show that alpha-lipoic acid increases blood flow to the nerves and enhances the conduction of nerve impulses. These effects may make alpha-lipoic acid suitable for the treatment of numbness, tingling and other symptoms of nerve damage from any cause, not only diabetes.

Alpha-lipoic acid also benefits the liver, protecting it against damage from free radicals and helping it to eliminate toxins from the body. It is sometimes used to treat hepatitis, cirrhosis and other liver ailments, as well as in cases of poisoning by lead or other heavy metals or by industrial chemicals such as carbon tetrachloride.

✳ **ADDITIONAL BENEFITS:** Alpha-lipoic acid may have other potential medicinal uses, but more research is needed. Some compelling studies in animals show that it can prevent cataracts from forming. Other animal experiments suggest that it may improve memory (making it beneficial in cases of Alzheimer's disease, for example) and protect brain cells against damage caused by an insufficient supply of blood to the brain – the result of surgery or stroke, for instance.

Some evidence indicates that alpha-lipoic acid's antioxidant properties make it effective in the suppression of viral reproduction. In one study, alpha-lipoic acid supplements were shown to boost the immune system and liver function in a majority of patients infected with AIDS. It may also help in the fight against cancer, especially the forms of the disease thought to be related to free-radical damage. There is evidence, too, that alpha-lipoic acid may help to slow the development of atherosclerosis, for which people with diabetes are at higher risk. Other studies are investigating the effectiveness of alpha-lipoic acid in Alzheimer's disease and Parkinson's disease. Finally, as part of a general high-potency antioxidant formula, alpha-lipoic acid may prove effective against disorders ranging from chronic fatigue syndrome to psoriasis, which may be aggravated, in part, by free-radical damage.

How to take it

▢ **DOSAGE:** *To treat specific disorders*: Alpha-lipoic acid is usually taken in doses of 100 to 200 mg three times a day. *For general antioxidant support*: Lower doses of 50 to 150 mg a day may be used.

◉ **GUIDELINES FOR USE:** Supplements of alpha-lipoic acid can be taken with or without food.

Possible side effects

There have been no reports of serious side effects in people taking alpha-lipoic acid. Occasionally the supplement may produce a mild upset stomach, and in rare cases allergic skin rashes have occurred. If side effects appear, lower the dose or stop using the supplement.

RECENT FINDINGS

In a study of people suffering from diabetic nerve damage, 328 patients were given 100 mg, 600 mg or 1200 mg of alpha-lipoic acid a day over a three-week period. Patients receiving 600 mg reported the most significant reduction in pain and numbness compared with the other groups.

—◆◆◆—

Alpha-lipoic acid may also benefit the 25% of diabetes sufferers at risk of sudden death from nerve-related heart damage. After four months of taking 800 mg of alpha-lipoic acid a day, these patients showed a notable improvement in heart function.

—◆◆◆—

A study of ageing mice indicated that alpha-lipoic acid improved long-term memory, possibly by preventing damage to brain cells by free radicals.

DID YOU KNOW?

Doctors have used an injectable form of alpha-lipoic acid to save the lives of people who became ill after eating poisonous amanita mushrooms picked in the wild.

Amino acids

The proteins in food and in the human body are combinations of chemical units called amino acids. A diet deficient in even one amino acid can have a damaging effect on health. Supplements may be needed to help the body to work more efficiently and to treat disease.

Common uses

- Treatment of heart disease.
- Lowering of blood pressure.
- Boosting immune function.
- Relieving some nervous disorders.

Forms

- Capsule
- Liquid
- Powder
- Tablet

What they are

Every cell in the body needs and uses amino acids. When you eat a meal, your digestive system breaks down the protein from foods into separate amino acids, which are then recombined to create the specific types of protein required by the body. (Each cell is programmed to produce exactly the right combination for its needs.) There are two types of amino acid: non-essential and essential. The body can manufacture non-essential amino acids but must obtain essential amino acids from foods. Non-essential amino acids include alanine, arginine, asparagine, aspartic acid, cysteine, glutamic acid, glutamine, glycine, proline, serine, taurine and tyrosine. Essential amino acids include histidine, isoleucine, leucine, lysine, methionine, phenylalanine, threonine, tryptophan and valine.

What they do

Amino acids are needed to maintain and repair muscles, tendons, skin, ligaments, organs, glands, nails and hair. They also assist in the production of hormones (such as insulin), neurotransmitters (message-carrying chemicals within the brain), various body fluids, and enzymes that trigger bodily functions.

Though the major cause of an amino acid deficiency is poor diet (particularly a diet low in protein), amino acids may also be affected by infection, trauma, stress, medication, age and chemical imbalances within the body. Nutritionally aware doctors may suggest a blood test to determine whether a patient has a deficiency. Amino acid supplements can compensate for deficiencies and can also be taken therapeutically to alleviate a number of health problems.

✪ **MAJOR BENEFITS:** Various amino acids, and their by-products, are very effective in the treatment of heart disease. Highly concentrated in the cells of the heart muscle, carnitine – a substance similar to an amino acid that the body produces from lysine – strengthens the heart, aids the

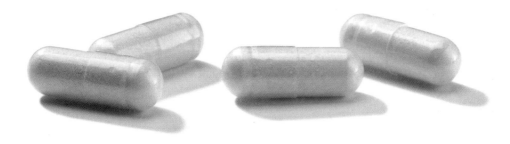

recovery of people who have suffered heart failure and can improve the chances of surviving a heart attack. As it is also involved in fat metabolism, carnitine may help to lower high levels of triglycerides (blood fats related to cholesterol). Arginine, a non-essential amino acid, reduces the risk of heart attack and stroke by widening blood vessels and lowering blood pressure; it can also ease the symptoms and pains of angina. Taurine treats heart failure and lowers high blood pressure by balancing the blood's sodium-to-potassium ratio and by regulating excessive activity of the central nervous system.

N-acetylcysteine (NAC), a by-product of cysteine that is more easily absorbed than cysteine, stimulates the body's production of antioxidants and may itself be an antioxidant. As such it aids in the repair of cell damage and boosts the immune system. NAC also thins the mucus of chronic bronchitis and has been used to protect the liver in overdoses of acetaminophen (Tylenol). It may also relieve disorders involving damage to brain or nerve cells, such as multiple sclerosis.

✳ **ADDITIONAL BENEFITS:** Concentrated in the cells of the digestive tract, glutamine soothes irritable bowel syndrome and diverticular disorders and helps to heal ulcers. By enhancing the production of certain brain chemicals, taurine may be a boon to people with epilepsy. It is also a key element in bile and may prevent gallstones. People with diabetes can benefit from taurine because it facilitates the body's use of insulin.

Carnitine feeds the muscles by making it possible for them to burn fat for energy. Lysine is one of the most effective treatments for cold sores and is also useful for shingles and mouth ulcers. (Arginine, on the other hand, can trigger outbreaks of cold sores or genital herpes.)

How to take them

⬛ **DOSAGE:** For the recommended dose of a particular amino acid supplement, refer to the appropriate ailment in the section Protecting Your Health. If you use an individual amino acid for longer than a month, take it with a mixed amino acid complex – a supplement that contains a variety of amino acids – to ensure that you are receiving adequate, balanced amounts of all the amino acids.

◉ **GUIDELINES FOR USE:** Amino acid supplements are more effective when they do not have to compete with the amino acids present in high-protein foods. For this reason, take the supplements at least 1½ hours before or after meals – the best times are probably first thing in the morning or at bedtime.

Individual amino acid supplements should not be used for longer than three months except under the supervision of a doctor familiar with their use. Take mixed amino acid supplements on an empty stomach and at a different time of day from when you take the individual supplement.

Possible side effects

As long as they are taken in the recommended amounts, amino acid supplements have no side effects. High doses of certain amino acids, however, may be toxic and induce nausea, vomiting or diarrhoea.

RECENT FINDINGS

In an Italian study involving 84 healthy older adults with the onset of fatigue following slight physical activity, 30 days of supplementation with carnitine improved mental and physical fatigue scores and increased total muscle mass. It also reduced total cholesterol, LDL cholesterol and triglyceride levels.

———

Researchers at Stanford University found that arginine supplements may reduce the tendency for blood platelets to stick to each other and to artery walls, and so prevent clots that cause heart attacks and strokes. Arginine particularly helps people with high cholesterol levels, who have stickier platelets than those with normal cholesterol.

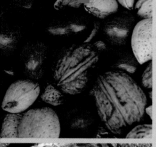
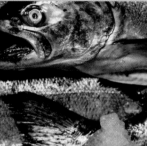
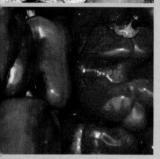

Antioxidants are substances in food used by the body as protection against free radicals, molecules produced during normal metabolism which can wreak havoc if they proliferate in an uncontrolled way as a result of illness, ageing or overexposure to toxins or the sun.

HOW FREE RADICALS CAUSE DAMAGE

Free radicals are highly unstable and quickly react with nearby molecules, setting off a process called oxidation which can have harmful effects on the body.

■ If free radicals oxidise DNA (the body's genetic code) in the nucleus of a cell, the reaction can cause cell mutations, which may initiate cancer.

■ The oxidation of cholesterol particles in the blood can trigger the build-up of fatty deposits in the arteries and lead to heart disease or stroke.

■ Free radicals have also been associated with cataracts, immune deficiency, arthritis and premature ageing, and their role in these conditions is still the subject of extensive research.

THE ROLE OF ANTIOXIDANTS

The body produces its own antioxidants, which neutralise the effects of free radicals, but vitamins, minerals and compounds known as phytochemicals in plant foods provide a valuable extra supply, so additional dietary sources are essential for the maintenance of good health. The table opposite lists the antioxidant vitamins and minerals as well as their food sources, and gives the officially recommended daily intakes, or RNIs (see page 26). In some cases the RNI is adequate for maintaining good health; in others the suggested optimum intake is higher. Even more doses may be recommended during illness or when diet has been inadequate.

■ A well-balanced multivitamin and multimineral formulation will supply enough mineral antioxidants, but extra supplies of vitamins C and E are required for optimum nutrition.

■ Other supplements can help to ease symptoms of certain illnesses. Coenzyme Q_{10}, for example, may be helpful for heart disease sufferers, or alpha-lipoic acid for those with diabetic neuropathy or AIDS.

■ Antioxidant phytochemicals can be taken as supplements.

■ Studies suggest that green tea extract, grapeseed extract and flavonoid preparations such as rutin can reduce the risk of cancer and heart disease.

■ Some phytochemicals seem to favour specific types of tissue. Extracts of bilberry are rich in anthocyanosides (flavonoid pigments), which improve the health of the retina of the eye.

■ Antioxidants in ginkgo extracts are effective in enhancing cerebral circulation and correcting memory loss.

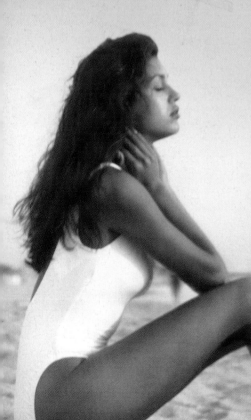

ANTIOXIDANT VITAMINS AND MINERALS

VITAMINS	ANTIOXIDANT EFFECTS	FOOD SOURCES	RECOMMENDED DAILY INTAKE (RNI)	SUGGESTED OPTIMUM DAILY INTAKE
Vitamin A, as retinol or as carotenoids	Diets high in carotenoids (some of which the body can convert into vitamin A) are linked with a reduced risk of some cancers; preliminary findings suggest that two carotenoids, lutein and zeaxanthin, may protect against age-related macular degeneration, a common cause of blindness in adults.	**Retinol**: animal foods such as liver, oily fish, eggs, milk, cheese and butter. **Carotenoids**: brightly coloured plant foods such as carrots, broccoli, dark green leafy vegetables, sweet red peppers, pumpkins, man-goes, canteloupe melons and dried apricots.	700 mcg for men; 600 mcg for women. Caretonoids: no RNI.	Supple-mentation not advised. Mixed caretonoids: 15 mg (see page 48)
Vitamin C	Scavenges for free radicals and regenerates the antioxidant potential of vitamin E after it has reacted with free radicals.	Citrus fruit, kiwi fruit, soft fruit such as blackcurrants and strawberries; potatoes, green and red peppers, tomatoes, bean sprouts and green leafy vegetables.	40 mg (80 mg for smokers)	200 mg (see page 162)
Vitamin E	Helps to prevent oxidation by free radicals of polyunsaturated fatty acids in cell membranes; the more polyunsaturated fats you eat, the more vitamin E you need to protect them from oxidation.	Vegetable oils such as sunflower and nut oils, margarine, almonds, hazelnuts, sunflower seeds, tuna, salmon, avocados.	No RNI; safe intake 10 mg, depending on intake of poly-unsaturated fat	100 mg (see page 166)
MINERALS				
Copper	Present in many enzymes that protect against free radical damage; required for healthy bone growth, for connective tissue formation, and to aid iron absorption from food.	Shellfish, liver, nuts, mushrooms and whole-grain cereals.	1.2 mg	RNI is adequate (see page 62)
Manganese	Present in enzymes that protect against free radical damage.	Nuts, brown rice, whole-grain bread, pulses and cereals; levels of manganese in plant foods depend on the amounts contained in the soil in which they are grown.	No RNI; safe intake 1.4 mg	
Selenium	Present in the enzyme that protects DNA against free radical damage; deficiency increases the risk of prostate cancer.	Brazil nuts, meat and offal, seafood and seaweed; avocados, whole grains and sunflower seeds also contain selenium, although levels depend on the amounts in the soil in which they were grown.	75 mcg for men; 60 mcg for women	RNI is adequate (see page 146)
Zinc	Present in enzymes that protect against free radical damage.	Shellfish (particularly oysters), lean meat, poultry, eggs and dairy products, pumpkin seeds, sunflower seeds, nuts and whole grains.	9.5 mg for men; 7 mg for women	RNI is adequate (see page 174)

Artichoke

Cynara scolymus

Artichoke's benefits were first documented by a pupil of Aristotle in the 4th century BC. The plant extract has long been popular in Germany for its positive dietary effects. It can bolster the actions of the gall bladder and liver, aid digestion and help to control cholesterol levels.

Common uses

- *Promotes healthy functioning of the gall bladder and liver.*
- *Improves digestion.*
- *Maintains and lowers levels of cholesterol.*
- *May help to control blood sugar levels, which is particularly important for diabetics.*

Forms

- Capsule
- Juice

CAUTION!

- If you are suffering from obstructive gall bladder disease, consult your doctor before taking artichoke extract because it increases bile secretion.

- A very small minority of people are allergic to artichoke and artichoke extract.

REMINDER: If you have a medical condition, consult your doctor before taking supplements.

What it is

Artichoke is a member of the botanical family that includes milk thistle, daisy and sunflower. Growing up to 2 metres in height, it is crowned with a large purple and green flower head. The young, unopened flower heads are cooked and the fleshy bases of the bracts, together with the receptacle, or 'heart', are eaten as a delicacy.

Also known as globe artichoke, the plant should not be confused with Jerusalem artichoke, the edible root vegetable. However, the globe artichoke is thought to have evolved from the cardoon that is grown in Mediterranean countries, and which has very similar medicinal qualities to the artichoke. The leaves of the globe artichoke contain several substances that have beneficial health effects when consumed at the recommended levels. They include cynarin (the key, active component) and various flavonoids, particularly luteolin.

What it does

Although artichoke leaf extract has been popular in Germany for some time, its benefits have only recently been recognised in the UK. Laboratory studies in Germany have shown it to be useful in the protection and regeneration of the liver following intoxication.

Scientific research dating back to 1933 shows that artichoke stimulates the production of bile from the liver, which then passes into the duodenum. This effect accounts for the successful use of the

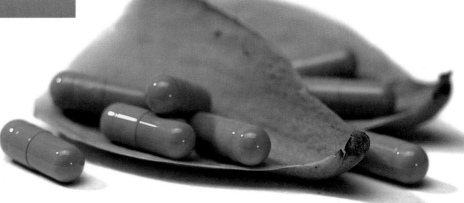

Artichoke supplements are made from the plant's leaves, and the edible bracts around the flower head (shown here) can help to control blood sugar levels.

herb in the treatment of people with impaired digestion of fat. Work undertaken as early as the 1930s showed that artichoke leaf extract was able to reduce blood cholesterol levels in patients with raised values. These findings have been confirmed by recent research, and one study has found that, while levels of LDL ('bad') cholesterol were lowered, there was a slight increase in levels of HDL ('good') cholesterol. It would seem that these cholesterol-lowering properties of artichoke extract are due to its content of luteolin, which inhibits the synthesis of cholesterol by the liver.

✳ **Major benefits:** Cynarin and the flavonoids of artichoke, including luteolin, are powerful antioxidants that can help to prevent cell damage in the liver, protect the body from damage by the unstable oxygen molecules known as free radicals, and hence help to fight disease. Several clinical studies have shown the extract to alleviate digestive disorders, such as abdominal pain, nausea and flatulence.

Artichoke contains inulin, a polysaccharide that slows down the rate at which the body digests food. This property means that, when eaten as a vegetable, artichoke may help to control blood sugar levels after meals, which makes it particularly useful for diabetics. People with high cholesterol levels may also benefit from the extract, which can reduce the synthesis of cholesterol in the liver.

✳ **Additional benefits:** Artichoke leaf has been traditionally used for its cleansing and detoxifying action in the treatment of gout, arthritis and rheumatism. Also, its diuretic action may help to alleviate urinary tract problems. Research is under way into other possible benefits, including its value for people suffering from irritable bowel syndrome. A recent study found significant reduction in the severity of symptoms in this condition.

How to take it

🖉 **Dosage:** *For improved digestion, liver function and cholesterol levels*: Take two 320 mg capsules daily. *For improved digestion at times of high fat intake*: Take up to six 320 mg capsules daily either at the same time or at different times during the day.

◉ **Guidelines for use:** Take capsules with or immediately after a meal and swallow them whole with cold liquid. If you suffer from gall bladder obstruction problems, consult your doctor before using artichoke. Anyone with an allergy to plants in the daisy family may experience an allergic reaction and should discontinue use at once.

Possible side effects

Many studies have confirmed that artichoke leaf extract is very well tolerated by most people, even after continuous long-term use. When taken as a food, artichoke presents minimal risks, but in a small minority of people it may cause side effects such as flatulence and mild gastrointestinal problems.

RECENT FINDINGS

A 1998 study of people with digestive problems showed that 85% experienced an improvement in their health from taking artichoke leaf extract. After the patients had taken five capsules a day for an average of 23 weeks their symptoms – which included nausea, flatulence, bloating, abdominal pain and fat intolerance – were all dramatically reduced.

A recent Germany study involving 553 people aged 20-87 found that artichoke extract had a beneficial effect on blood cholesterol levels. After six weeks of treatment the subjects found that their blood cholesterol levels had dropped by an average of 11.5%.

DID YOU KNOW?

The ancient Greeks introduced globe artichoke into Europe from North Africa. It has long been popular in France, where it is served in salads or as an appetiser.

Astragalus

Astragalus membranaceus

For more than 2000 years astragalus has played an integral part in the traditional medicine of China, where it is used to balance the life force, or *qi*. The Chinese name for the herb is *huang qi*, meaning 'yellow leader', reflecting its therapeutic importance.

Common uses

- *Enhances immunity.*
- *Helps to fight respiratory infections.*
- *Bolsters the immune system in people undergoing cancer treatment.*

Forms

- Capsule
- Dried herb/tea
- Tablet
- Tincture

CAUTION!

- **Pregnant or breastfeeding women should seek medical advice before using this herb.**

REMINDER: If you have a medical condition, consult your doctor before taking supplements.

What it is

Astragalus contains a variety of compounds that are known to stimulate the body's immune system, and in China this native plant has long been used both to prevent and to treat disease. Botanically, astragalus is related to liquorice and the pea. Although its sweet-smelling, pale yellow blossoms and delicate structure give the plant a frail appearance, it is actually a very hardy species. Medicinally, the most important part of the astragalus plant is its root, which is loaded with health-promoting substances including polysaccharides, a class of carbohydrate, that appear to be responsible for its immune-boosting effects. Astragalus is harvested when it is four to seven years old; after they have been sliced for use, its yellowish roots resemble the broad flat sticks that are used to hold ice-lollies.

What it does

A tonic in the true sense of the word, astragalus has the capacity to enhance overall health by improving resistance to disease, increasing stamina and vitality, and promoting general well-being. It also acts as an antioxidant, helping the human body to correct or prevent cell damage caused by free radicals. It may also have antiviral and antibiotic properties. Supplements derived from the herb can be safely used in combination with conventional medicines.

PREVENTION: Astragalus is particularly effective in fighting off colds, flu, bronchitis and sinus infections because it inhibits viruses from establishing themselves in the respiratory system. Like echinacea, astragalus can destroy harmful bacteria as soon as the symptoms of respiratory infection start to appear. If an illness does develop, astragalus can shorten its duration and reduce its severity. People who frequently suffer from respiratory illnesses should consider using

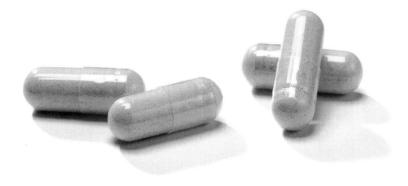

astragalus on a regular basis to prevent recurrences. It also helps to minimise the detrimental effects on health caused by excessive stress.

⁂ **ADDITIONAL BENEFITS:** Astragalus is widely used in China to rebuild the immune systems of cancer patients who have received radiotherapy or chemotherapy – a practice that is also gaining popularity in the West. The herb increases the body's production of T-cells, macrophages, natural killer cells, interferon and other immune cells. Astragalus may also protect bone marrow from the immunosuppressive effects of chemotherapy, radiotherapy, toxins and viruses. The herb, which stimulates the immune response, is a possible treatment for people infected with HIV, the virus that causes AIDS.

In addition, astragalus widens blood vessels and increases blood flow, which makes it useful in controlling excessive perspiration (such as night sweats) and lowering blood pressure. Research has also shown that astragalus can have beneficial effects on the heart and it can enhance the motility of sperm.

How to take it

⬛ **DOSAGE:** *For strengthening the immune system*: Take 200 mg of astragalus extract once or twice a day for three weeks, then alternate, in three-week stints, with echinacea, cat's claw and pau d'arco. *For acute bronchitis*: Take 200 mg four times a day until the symptoms ease. Choose a product that contains a standardised extract of astragalus with 0.5% glucosides and 70% polysaccharides.

⬛ **GUIDELINES FOR USE:** Astragalus can be taken at any time during the day, with or without meals.

Possible side effects

Remarkably, even after thousands of years of use in China, there are few (if any) negative reports associated with the medicinal use of astragalus.

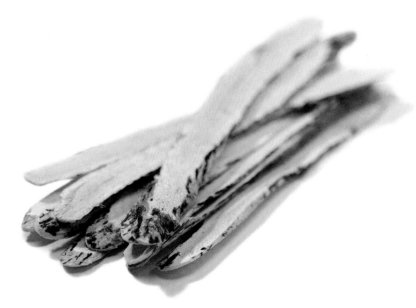

Bee products

Although many intriguing claims have been made for the healing powers of bee products, there is little evidence to support most of them. But bee pollen, royal jelly and propolis are popular nutritional supplements, and continue to be the subject of scientific studies.

Common uses

- *May relieve symptoms of hay fever.*
- *Propolis helps to heal skin abrasions.*

Forms

- Capsule
- Cream
- Dried and fresh pollen
- Liquid
- Lozenge
- Powder
- Softgel
- Tablet

CAUTION!

- Asthmatics or people who are allergic to bee stings should be very careful when using bee products; they should avoid royal jelly entirely.

REMINDER: *If you have a medical condition, consult your doctor before taking supplements.*

What they are

There are three types of bee products available in health-food shops: bee pollen, propolis and royal jelly. Bee pollen, which comes from flowers, is distinct from the airborne pollen produced by grasses that often causes hay fever. After bees have gathered pollen, they compress it into pellets, which can be collected from their hives. (A second type of pollen, also sold as bee pollen, is collected directly from plants.) Bee pollen contains protein, B vitamins, carbohydrates and various enzymes. Propolis – also called bee glue – is a sticky resin that bees collect from the buds of pine trees and use to repair cracks in their hives. Royal jelly is a milky-white substance produced by the salivary glands of worker bees as a food source for the queen bee. The specialised nutritional content of royal jelly may account for the fertility, large size and longevity of the queen.

What they do

Bee products, especially bee pollen, have been touted as virtual cure-alls. Proponents assert that, among other things, these products slow ageing, improve athletic performance, boost immunity, contribute to weight loss, fight bacteria and alleviate the symptoms of allergies and hay fever. Although bee pollen shows some promise in treating allergies, and propolis may be effective as a salve for cuts and bruises, the scant research that has been conducted into bee products does not support the extravagant claims made for them.

✪ **MAJOR BENEFITS:**
Bee pollen may help to prevent the sneezing, runny nose, watery eyes and other symptoms suffered by people susceptible to seasonal allergies triggered by flower pollen. Some scientists believe that ingesting small amounts of pollen can desensitise an individual to its allergenic compounds, much as allergy inoculations do. The theory is that, when

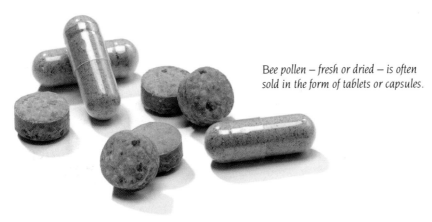

Bee pollen – fresh or dried – is often sold in the form of tablets or capsules.

exposed to even a tiny amount of pollen, the human immune system produces antibodies whose task is to provide protection against the extreme reaction that causes classic allergy symptoms. Tests of this theory continue, but meanwhile bee pollen poses no apparent danger to most people. Some advocates maintain that, for best results, sufferers need to use bee pollen from a local source, in order to desensitise them to the flower pollens in their own particular environment.

❋ **ADDITIONAL BENEFITS:** Propolis may have a role as a skin softener or a wound healer. Although it contains antibacterial compounds, research has shown that these are not as effective as standard antibiotics or over-the-counter antibiotic ointments in fighting infection.

The fact that royal jelly enhances the growth, fertility and longevity of queen bees has led many people to think that it will do the same for humans. There is no evidence to support this view, but royal jelly has long been highly regarded in traditional Chinese medicine for its efficacy in restoring strength after illness.

How to take them

☑ **DOSAGE:** The amount of bee pollen needed to relieve allergy symptoms varies from person to person. In general, start with a few granules a day and increase the dose gradually until you reach 1 to 3 rounded teaspoons a day.

◉ **GUIDELINES FOR USE:** Before the hay-fever season begins, take very small amounts of bee pollen each day – a few granules or a portion of a tablet. If you do not suffer any adverse reaction, increase the dosage slowly until you experience relief from allergy symptoms. Bee-pollen supplements should be consumed with plenty of water; you can also mix dried or fresh pollen with juice or sprinkle it over food.

Possible side effects

Some individuals have allergic reactions to bee pollen, which can include asthma, eczema and a runny nose. Start by taking a small amount so that you can determine if you are susceptible. If you develop a rash, an itchy throat, skin flushing, wheezing or headaches, stop using it immediately.

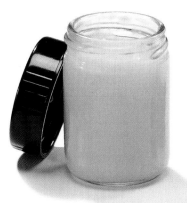
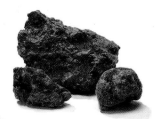
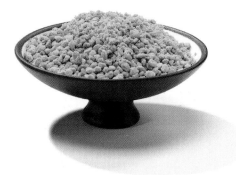

The three types of bee product on the market are royal jelly (left), the sticky resin called propolis (centre) and bee pollen (right).

Bilberry

Vaccinium myrtillus

During the Second World War, RAF pilots noted the curious fact that their night vision improved after eating bilberry jam. Their anecdotal reports stimulated scientific research into bilberry, which is now used to treat a wide range of visual disorders and other complaints.

Common uses

- *Maintains healthy vision as well as improving night vision and poor visual adaptation to bright light.*
- *Treats a wide array of eye disorders, including diabetic retinopathy, cataracts and macular degeneration.*
- *Relieves varicose veins and haemorrhoids, especially in pregnant women.*

Forms

- Capsule
- Dried herb/tea
- Softgel
- Tablet
- Tincture

What it is

Although the fruit of the bilberry bush has been eaten with pleasure since prehistoric times, its first recorded medicinal use was in the 16th century. Historically, dried berry or leaf preparations were recommended for the treatment of a variety of conditions, including scurvy (caused by vitamin C deficiency), urinary tract infections and kidney stones.

Bilberry is a short, shrubby perennial that grows in the forests and on the moors of northern Europe. Bushes of the sweet blue-black berries are also found in western Asia and the Rocky Mountains of North America. The health-promoting components of the ripe fruit consist primarily of flavonoid compounds known as anthocyanosides, and the modern medicinal form of bilberry is an extract containing a highly concentrated amount of these compounds.

What it does

Many of the medicinal qualities of bilberry derive from anthocyanosides, the plant's main constituents, which are potent antioxidants. These compounds help to counteract cell damage caused by the unstable oxygen molecules known as free radicals.

MAJOR BENEFITS: Bilberry extract is the leading herbal remedy for maintaining healthy vision and managing various eye disorders. In particular, bilberry helps the retina, the light-sensitive portion of the eye, to adapt properly to dark and light. It has been widely used to treat night blindness as well as poor vision resulting from daytime glare. With its ability to strengthen the tiny blood vessels called capillaries – and, in

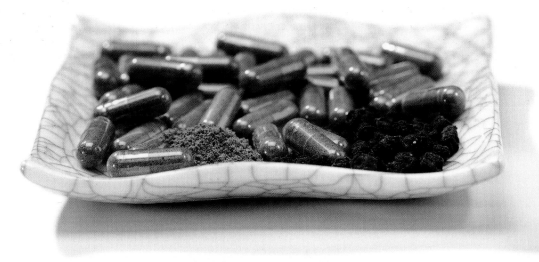

Bilberries, available in capsule form, provide a popular herbal remedy for a variety of eye disorders.

turn, facilitate the delivery of oxygen-rich blood to the eyes – bilberry may also play a significant role in preventing and treating degenerative diseases of the retina (retinopathy). In one study, 31 patients were treated with bilberry extract daily for four weeks. Use of the extract fortified the capillaries and reduced haemorrhaging in the eyes, especially in cases of diabetic retinopathy.

Bilberry is used to treat two leading causes of sight loss in older people: macular degeneration, a progressive disorder affecting the central part of the retina, and cataract, the loss of transparency in the lens of the eye. A study of 50 patients with age-related cataracts found that bilberry extract combined with vitamin E supplements inhibited cataract formation in almost all participants. Bilberry is known to strengthen collagen – the abundant protein that forms the 'backbone' of healthy connective tissue – which may make it valuable in the prevention and treatment of glaucoma, a disease caused by excessive pressure within the eye.

ADDITIONAL BENEFITS: As the anthocyanosides in bilberry improve the blood flow in capillaries as well as in larger blood vessels, bilberry in standardised extract form may be efficacious for people with poor circulation in their extremities. It is helpful in treating varicose veins and in easing the pain and burning of haemorrhoids, particularly during pregnancy when both these conditions can be very troublesome. People who bruise easily may also benefit from bilberry's effect on capillaries.

Although more research is needed, there are indications that the plant may have other medicinal uses. One study demonstrated that long-term use of bilberry extract improved the vision of normally short-sighted people – but how it produced this effect is unknown. Preliminary results from tests on women showed that bilberry helps to relieve menstrual cramps because anthocyanosides relax smooth muscle, including the uterus. Animal studies suggest that bilberry anthocyanosides may fight stomach ulcers and may also reduce levels of triglycerides (a type of fat) in the blood.

How to take it

DOSAGE: Normal doses range from 40 to 160 mg of bilberry extract two or three times a day. The lower dose is generally recommended for long-term use, including prevention of macular degeneration; higher doses – up to 320 mg a day – may be needed by people with diabetes.

GUIDELINES FOR USE: Bilberry can be taken with or without food. No adverse effects have been noted in pregnant or breastfeeding women who use the herb. In addition, there are no known adverse interactions with prescription or over-the-counter drugs.

Possible side effects

In therapeutic doses, bilberry appears to be very safe and has no known side effects, even when taken over a long period of time.

Biotin and pantothenic acid

These two B vitamins play a vital role in sustaining efficient metabolic function. Deficiencies are rare, but supplements can help in treating various disorders and may be useful for people whose diets include a lot of processed foods.

Common uses

Biotin
- *Promotes healthy nails and hair.*
- *Helps the body to use carbohydrates, fats and protein.*
- *May improve blood-sugar control in people with diabetes.*

Pantothenic acid
- *Promotes a healthy central nervous system.*
- *Helps the body to use carbohydrates, fats and protein.*
- *May alleviate chronic fatigue syndrome, migraines, indigestion and the symptoms of some allergies.*

Forms
- Capsule
- Liquid
- Softgel
- Tablet

CAUTION!

REMINDER: If you have a medical condition, consult your doctor before taking supplements.

What they are

Biotin and pantothenic acid are vitamins contained in many foods, so deficiencies are virtually non-existent. Biotin is also produced by intestinal bacteria, though the vitamin may be hard for the body to use in this form. Multivitamins and B-complex vitamins usually include biotin and pantothenic acid (also called vitamin B_5), and both are available as individual supplements. The main form of biotin is D-biotin. Pantothenic acid comes in two forms, pantethine and calcium pantothenate; the latter is suitable for most purposes and is less expensive than pantethine.

What they do

Both biotin and pantothenic acid are involved in the production of various enzymes and in the breaking down of carbohydrates, fats and protein from foods so that they can be used by the body. Biotin plays a special role in helping the body to use glucose, its basic fuel, as well as promoting healthy nails and hair. The body needs pantothenic acid to maintain proper communication between the brain and the nervous system and to produce certain stress hormones.

✴ **MAJOR BENEFITS:** Biotin supplements improve the quality of weak and brittle fingernails and help to slow down hair loss caused by a biotin deficiency. Pantothenic acid is used to manufacture stress hormones, and during long periods of emotional upset, depression or anxiety – which are generally accompanied by an overproduction of stress hormones – the body's need for the vitamin appears to increase. The stress caused by migraines or chronic fatigue syndrome, or by the challenge of giving up smoking, may be alleviated by pantothenic acid supplements. In combination with the B vitamins choline and thiamin, pantothenic acid can be an effective remedy for indigestion; it also relieves the nasal congestion caused by certain allergic reactions, such as hay fever.

✴ **ADDITIONAL BENEFITS:** Biotin in very high doses may benefit diabetics, increasing the body's response to insulin so that levels of blood sugar (glucose) stay low. It may protect against the nerve damage that can occur in diabetes. Diabetics should seek medical advice.

Biotin (left) and pantothenic acid (right) are important B vitamins.

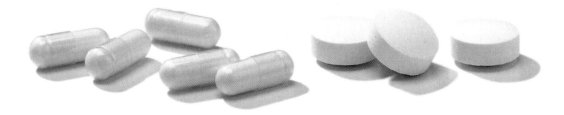

How much you need

There is no RDA for biotin or pantothenic acid, but 30 to 100 mcg of biotin and 4 to 7 mg of pantothenic acid a day appear to be enough to maintain healthy bodily functions. For the treatment of specific diseases or disorders, higher doses may be needed.

⊟ **IF YOU GET TOO LITTLE:** Deficiencies of biotin or pantothenic acid are virtually unknown in adults. Long-term use of antibiotics or anti-seizure medications, however, can lead to less-than-optimal levels of biotin.

⊞ **IF YOU GET TOO MUCH:** Although no serious adverse effects from high doses of biotin or pantothenic acid have been recorded, the daily recommended upper safe levels of, respectively, 900 mcg and 200 mg should not be exceeded.

How to take them

⊘ **DOSAGE:** *For hair and nails:* Take up to 900 mcg of biotin a day. *During periods of stress:* Take 100 mg of pantothenic acid a day as part of a vitamin B complex. *For migraines:* Take 100 mg of pantothenic acid twice a day. *For chronic fatigue syndrome:* Take 100 mg of pantothenic acid twice a day. *For chronic indigestion:* Take 100 mg of pantothenic acid twice a day along with 50 mg of thiamin first thing in the morning and 500 mg of choline three times a day. *For allergies:* Take 100 mg of pantothenic acid twice a day. *For diabetes:* Consult your doctor about taking high doses of biotin to relieve or even to prevent diabetic neuropathy.

⊕ **GUIDELINES FOR USE:** A multivitamin or a B-complex supplement will provide enough biotin and pantothenic acid for most people. Individual supplements are necessary only to treat specific disorders. In most cases, individual supplements should be taken with meals.

Other sources

Biotin is found in liver, soy products, nuts, oatmeal, rice, barley, legumes, cauliflower and whole wheat. Offal, fish, poultry, whole grains, yoghurt and legumes are the best sources of pantothenic acid.

Nuts such as sweet chestnuts are a useful natural source of biotin.

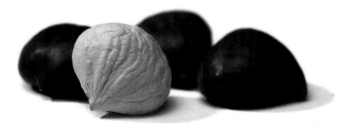

Black cohosh

The gnarled black root of the black cohosh plant was identified more than a century ago as the source of one of the most useful natural medicines for women. The name 'cohosh', derived from a Native American word for 'rough', refers to the twisted appearance of the root.

Cimicifuga racemosa

Common uses

- *Reduces menopausal symptoms, particularly hot flushes.*
- *Eases menstrual pain and associated conditions, such as PMS.*
- *Works as an anti-inflammatory; relieves muscle pain.*
- *Helps to clear mucous membranes and to relieve coughs.*

Forms

- Capsule
- Dried herb/tea
- Tablet
- Tincture

What it is

Long used to treat 'women's problems', the black cohosh plant grows up to 2½ metres high and is distinguished by its tall stalks of fluffy white flowers. Native to North America, this member of the buttercup family is also known as bugbane, squawroot or rattle root. However, its most common nickname, black snakeroot, describes its gnarled black root, the part of the plant that is used medicinally. Contained in the root is a complex mixture of natural chemicals, some as powerful as the most modern pharmaceuticals.

What it does

Traditionally, black cohosh has been prescribed to treat menstrual problems, pain after childbirth, nervous disorders and joint pain. Today the herb is recommended primarily for relief of the hot flushes that some women experience during the menopause.

✪ **MAJOR BENEFITS:** Black cohosh is an increasingly popular remedy for hot flushes, excessive sweating, vaginal dryness and other menopausal symptoms. Scientific study has shown that it can reduce levels of LH (luteinising hormone), which is produced by the brain's pituitary gland. The rise in LH that occurs during the menopause is thought to be one cause of hot flushes.

The root of black cohosh is dried, ground to a powder and sold as a supplement in capsule form.

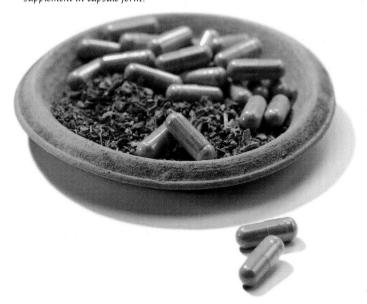

In addition, black cohosh contains phytoestrogens, plant compounds that have an effect similar to that of oestrogen produced by the body. Phytoestrogens bind themselves to hormone receptors in the breasts, uterus and elsewhere in the body, easing menopausal symptoms without increasing the risk of breast cancer, a possible side effect of hormone replacement therapy. Some phytoestrogens may even help to prevent breast cancer by inhibiting the body's own oestrogen from locking onto breast cells.

✳ **ADDITIONAL BENEFITS:** Black cohosh's antispasmodic properties mean that it has the power to alleviate menstrual cramps by increasing blood flow to the uterus and reducing the intensity of uterine contractions. This action also makes it useful during labour and after childbirth. Black cohosh 'evens out' hormone levels, offering possible benefits to women suffering from premenstrual syndrome (PMS), but chasteberry is probably more effective in relieving this condition.

Although these capabilities are less frequently noted, black cohosh has demonstrated some mildly sedative and anti-inflammatory effects, which may be particularly valuable in treating muscle aches as well as nerve-related pain caused by, for example, sciatica or neuralgia. It can help to clear mucus from the body and has been recommended for coughs. The herb has also been shown to be an effective treatment for tinnitus (ringing in the ears).

How to take it

🖉 **DOSAGE:** Look for capsules or tablets containing extracts that have been standardised to contain 2.5% of triterpenes, the active components in black cohosh. *For menopausal or* PMS *symptoms*: Take 40 mg of black cohosh extract twice a day. For PMS, begin treatment a week to 10 days before the start of your period. *For menstrual cramps*: Take 40 mg three or four times a day as needed.

◉ **GUIDELINES FOR USE:** Black cohosh can be taken at any time of day, but to reduce the chance of stomach upset you may prefer to take it with meals. Allow four to eight weeks to see its benefits. Many researchers recommend a six-month limit on taking black cohosh, though recent studies show that longer use seems to be safe and free of significant side effects.

Possible side effects

Though it has virtually no toxic effects, black cohosh may cause stomach upsets in certain people. One study suggested that it may induce slight weight gain and dizziness in some women. It may also lower blood pressure. A very high dose can cause nausea, vomiting, reduced pulse rate, heavy perspiration and headaches.

FACTS & TIPS

▪ Compresses soaked in black cohosh tea can be used to soothe sore muscles and aching joints. Boil the dried root in water for 20 to 30 minutes. Let the liquid cool a bit (it should still be hot, but not hot enough to burn your skin). Then apply the warm compress to the affected area and leave it there for about 20 minutes.

▪ Recent research suggests that black cohosh helps to relieve the menopausal symptoms of hot flushes and night sweats by acting on the receptors in the brain used to control body temperature, and not by influencing oestrogen.

Bromelain

A digestive enzyme with anti-inflammatory properties, bromelain is derived from the pineapple plant. It has been used since the 1950s for a wide variety of therapeutic purposes, relieving conditions from sports injuries to heart disease.

Common uses

- *Reduces pain and swelling caused by minor injuries.*
- *Aids healing of wounds and post-operative recovery.*
- *Reduces mucous congestion in bronchitis and sinusitis.*
- *Improves the effectiveness of some antibiotics.*
- *Helps in the digestion of protein.*

Form

- Tablet

What it is

Bromelain is a protein-digesting, milk-clotting enzyme found in fresh pineapple. The commercial supplement is usually obtained only from the pineapple stem, which is different from the enzyme in the fruit. It is produced mainly in Japan, Taiwan and Hawaii.

What it does

Bromelain is a powerful anti-inflammatory agent which can reduce pain and swelling and promote tissue repair. Its effectiveness is thought to spring from its interaction with hormone-like substances known as prostaglandins. Bromelain can inhibit the action of prostaglandins that cause pain and inflammation while promoting the formation of different, anti-inflammatory prostaglandins. It also stimulates the breakdown of fibrin, an insoluble protein that can be associated with fluid retention. Bromelain is unusual as a protein-digesting enzyme in that it bypasses the digestive tract to be absorbed intact.

MAJOR BENEFITS: Bromelain's anti-inflammatory action makes it useful in the treatment of the pain and swelling associated with sprains and muscle injuries as well as in the healing of wounds and burns. In one study involving 700 firemen with burns, those who took bromelain found that their injuries healed in half the time that they took to heal in those who were not given the enzyme.

Other evidence shows that bromelain helps to reduce the bruising and pain that can follow minor operations, especially in women who have had surgery after childbirth. When combined with another

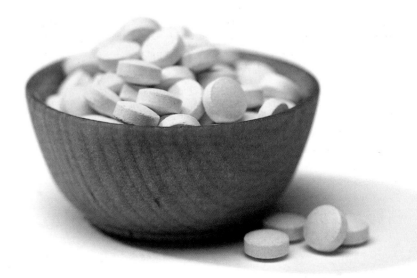

proteolytic enzyme called trypsin, bromelain may be effective against urinary tract infections. In a preliminary study 78% of sufferers said that their symptoms were eased by taking the enzyme combination. Taken together with papain, bromelain may also ease period pain by reducing spasms in the uterus.

✦ **ADDITIONAL BENEFITS:** By counteracting excessive stickiness of blood platelets the enzyme helps to combat cardiovascular disease, reducing the threat of thrombosis and the pain of angina, and relaxing arterial constriction. Angina sufferers who took between 1000 mg and 1400 mg of bromelain reported a disappearance of all their symptoms within a period of 4 to 90 days. (The length of time it took for the improvements to become evident was related to the severity of the patients' original symptoms.)

As a protein-digesting enzyme, bromelain may have an anticancer effect, but more evidence is needed. Also, it may boost the effectiveness of chemotherapy and possibly inhibit the growth of cancer cells. When taken orally, the enzyme has been shown to bring about the synthesis of anticancer compounds.

Bromelain appears to reduce the thickness of mucus, which may be helpful in the treatment of asthma or chronic bronchitis. It has also been shown to be effective in alleviating sinusitis. Other studies show that the enzyme can aid the absorption of antibiotics such as amoxicillin and penicillin, as well as assisting the absorption of curcumin, the active ingredient in turmeric. There is some evidence to suggest that, when used with papain, a proteolytic enzyme found in unripe papaya, bromelain may relieve painful menstrual periods.

As an anti-inflammatory, bromelain may be useful for relieving rheumatoid arthritis. In a preliminary study 73% of patients given a supplement for periods of between three weeks and 13 months reported good to excellent results. Since bromelain can reduce the swelling and bruising that may follow an operation, while leaving the blood-clotting process unaffected, it may sometimes be given to patients who are about to undergo liposuction.

How to take it

▢ **DOSAGE:** A typical recommended dose of bromelain is between 250 mg and 500 mg three times a day.

◖ **GUIDELINES FOR USE:** Bromelain should generally be taken on an empty stomach, but when used as a digestive aid it should be taken with food, especially to assist in the digestion of fatty or high-protein meals. For the relief of swelling or inflammation continue to take the supplement until symptoms subside.

Possible side effects

Even when bromelain is taken in very large doses, side effects are extremely rare. Some people with particular sensitivity may experience allergic reactions and skin irritation. There has been a preliminary report of increased heart rate associated with the use of the enzyme.

Calcium

Renowned for its importance in combating osteoporosis, calcium is now thought to have a role in lowering blood pressure and preventing colon cancer. But modern diets are often severely lacking in calcium; many adults get only half the daily recommended quantities of the mineral.

Common uses

- *Maintains healthy bones and teeth.*
- *Helps to prevent progressive bone loss and osteoporosis.*
- *Aids heart and muscle contraction, nerve impulses and blood clotting.*
- *Eases indigestion.*

Forms

- Capsule
- Liquid
- Powder
- Softgel
- Tablet

CAUTION!

- People with thyroid or kidney disease should seek medical advice before taking calcium.
- Calcium may interact with some drugs, notably the tetracycline antibiotics.

REMINDER: If you have a medical condition, consult your doctor before taking supplements.

What it is

An essential constituent of bones and teeth, calcium is also required for bodily functions such as blood clotting and muscle contraction. Eating enough calcium-rich foods may be difficult, but supplements can prevent the development of a deficiency. The most common forms are calcium carbonate, calcium citrate, calcium citrate malate, calcium gluconate, calcium phosphate and calcium lactate. The amount of elemental – or pure – calcium in a supplement varies from compound to compound. Calcium carbonate (used in antacids to relieve indigestion) provides 40% elemental calcium, while calcium gluconate supplies 9%: the lower the calcium content, the more pills needed to meet recommended amounts.

What it does

Most of the body's calcium is stored in the bones and teeth, where it provides structure and strength. The small amount circulating in the bloodstream helps to move nutrients across cell membranes and plays a role in producing the hormones and enzymes that regulate digestion and metabolism. Calcium is also needed for normal communication between nerve cells and for blood clotting, wound healing and muscle contraction. To have enough of the mineral available in the blood to perform vital functions, the body will steal it from the bones. Over time, too many calcium 'withdrawals' leave bones porous and fragile. Only an adequate daily calcium intake will maintain healthy levels in the blood – and provide enough extra for the bones to absorb as a reserve.

PREVENTION: Getting enough calcium throughout life is a central factor in preventing osteoporosis, the bone-thinning disease that leads to a higher risk of hip and vertebra fractures, spinal deformities and loss of height. The body is best equipped to absorb calcium and build up bone mass before the age of 35, but several studies have shown that even people aged over 65 can maintain bone density and reduce the risk of fractures by taking calcium supplements and eating calcium-rich foods.

ADDITIONAL BENEFITS: By limiting the irritating effects of bile acids in the colon, calcium may reduce the incidence of colon cancer. Calcium

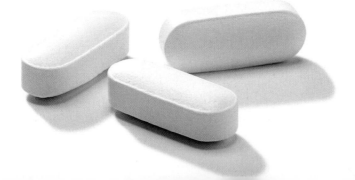

may also be useful for treating the symptoms of premenstrual syndrome and period pain. A trial of 497 women with PMS found that 100 mg of calcium daily for three months reduced symptoms significantly more than a placebo.

How much you need

In the UK the current recommended daily target of calcium, for both men and women, is 700 mg, with no extra amount recommended for pregnant women. But the equivalent recommendation in the USA is 1000 mg for men and women aged from 19 to 50 and 1200 mg for those from 50 to 70.

⊟ **IF YOU GET TOO LITTLE:** A prolonged calcium deficiency can lead to bone abnormalities, such as osteoporosis. Low levels of calcium in the blood can cause muscle spasms.

⊞ **IF YOU GET TOO MUCH:** A daily calcium intake of 1500 mg from supplements appears to be safe. However, taking calcium supplements may impair the body's ability to absorb zinc, iron and magnesium. Very high doses of calcium from supplements could lead to kidney stones. If calcium carbonate supplements cause flatulence or constipation they can be replaced by calcium citrate.

How to take it

▨ **DOSAGE:** Ensure that you get the recommended amount of 700 mg of elemental calcium a day from foods, supplements or both. When taking calcium, it may be advisable to take magnesium supplements as well, in a ratio of 1 to 2. So if you take 500 mg of supplemental calcium, take 250 mg of magnesium with it.

◉ **GUIDELINES FOR USE:** To enhance efficient absorption, split up your supplement dose so that you do not consume more than 600 mg of calcium at any one time. Always take the supplements with food. Those containing calcium citrate or malate are more easily absorbed by the body than those containing calcium carbonate.

Other sources

The most plentiful sources of calcium are dairy products, such as milk, yoghurt and cheese. Low-fat or fat-free varieties contain slightly more calcium than the full-fat types. Orange juice fortified with calcium malate, tinned salmon and sardines (eaten with the soft bones), broccoli and almonds are good non-dairy sources.

DID YOU KNOW?

Calcium cannot be absorbed without sufficient quantities of vitamin D, which is made by the skin in response to sunlight.

FACTS & TIPS

■ Avoid calcium supplements made from dolomite, oyster shells or bonemeal; they may contain high levels of lead.

■ The body's ability to convert sunlight to vitamin D declines with age, so it is advisable to include 10 mcg in your daily diet. This may mean taking a supplement, such as one containing both calcium and vitamin D.

■ Your body can absorb only a fraction of the calcium in spinach. Spinach contains high levels of oxalates, which lock up the calcium and limit the amount available to the body. Oxalates do not interfere with calcium absorption from other foods eaten at the same time, however.

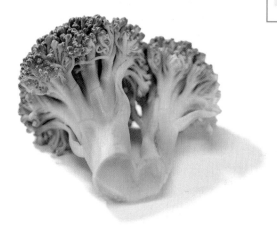

A 100 gram serving of boiled broccoli provides only one twentieth of an adult's daily calcium needs.

Carotenoids

The pigments that give some vegetables and fruits their rich red, orange and yellow colours are called carotenoids. These natural antioxidants are also potent disease fighters. A popular way of enjoying the benefits of carotenoids is by taking a combination supplement.

Common uses

- *May lower the risk of certain types of cancers, including prostate and lung cancer.*
- *May provide protection against heart disease.*
- *Slow the development of macular degeneration.*
- *Enhance immunity.*

Forms

- Capsule
- Softgel
- Tablet

CAUTION!

- High doses of carotenoids should be avoided in pregnancy.

REMINDER: If you have a medical condition, consult your doctor before taking supplements.

What they are

Although more than 600 carotenoid pigments have been identified in foods, it appears that only six of them are used in significant ways by the blood or tissues of the body. Apart from beta-carotene, which is probably the best-known carotenoid, these are alpha-carotene, cryptoxanthin, lycopene, lutein and zeaxanthin.

Carotenoids are found in a wide variety of fruits and vegetables, but the foods that represent the most concentrated sources may not be part of your daily diet. Alpha-carotene is found in carrots and pumpkin; lycopene is abundant in red fruits, such as watermelon, red grapefruit, guava and, in particular, cooked tomatoes. Lutein and zeaxanthin are plentiful in dark green vegetables, pumpkin and red peppers; and cryptoxanthin is present in mangoes, oranges and peaches. To prevent certain diseases it may be advisable to choose supplements that provide a mixture of the six key carotenoids.

What they do

The primary benefit of carotenoids lies in their antioxidant effect – protecting the cells of the body from damage by unstable oxygen molecules called free radicals. Although carotenoids are similar to one another, each acts on a specific type of bodily tissue. In addition, alpha-carotene and cryptoxanthin can be converted into vitamin A in the body, but not to the same extent as beta-carotene.

⊙ **PREVENTION:** Carotenoids may guard against certain types of cancer, apparently by limiting the abnormal growth of cells. Lycopene, for instance, appears to inhibit the development of prostate cancer. Researchers at Harvard University found that men who ate ten or more servings a week of tomato-based foods – tomatoes are the richest dietary source of lycopene – cut their risk of prostate cancer by nearly 45%. Lycopene may also be effective against cancers of the stomach and digestive tract. Studies show that high intakes of alpha-carotene, lutein and zeaxanthin decrease the risk of lung cancer, and that cryptoxanthin and alpha-carotene lower the risk of cervical cancer. Carotenoids may also fight heart disease. In a survey of 1300 elderly people, those who

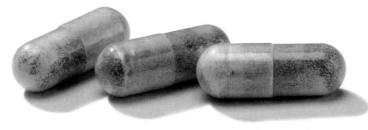

Though capsules of individual carotenoids such as lycopene (left) are available, it is even more beneficial to take a mixed carotenoid supplement.

consumed the greatest amount of carotenoid-rich foods were shown to have half the risk of developing heart disease, and a 75% lower chance of heart attack, than those who ate the least amount of these foods. This was true even after taking account of other risk factors for heart disease, such as smoking and high cholesterol levels. Scientists believe that all carotenoids, particularly alpha-carotene and lycopene, block the formation of LDL ('bad') cholesterol, which can lead to heart attacks and other cardiovascular problems.

✠ **ADDITIONAL BENEFITS:** Lutein and zeaxanthin are important for eye health, *see page* 118. Other carotenoids may also help protect the eye, reducing the risk of diseases such as cataracts. Studies have identified protective effects for lycopene against oxidative damage in the human lens and reduced incidence of cataract in test animals. A survey of 372 older people also found that the risk of cortical cataract was lowest in the people with the highest blood concentrations of lycopene.

A recent study found that increasing lycopene intake from tomato paste to 16mg/day over a 10-week period offered significant protection against sunburn following UV radiation, although the protective effects appear to develop slowly. Lycopene should not be used as a substitute for protective sunscreens.

How to take them

☑ **DOSAGE:** If you do not eat a wide variety of carotenoid-rich foods, choose a supplement that contains a mixture of carotenoids – alpha-carotene, beta-carotene, cryptoxanthin, lycopene, lutein and zeaxanthin.

◉ **GUIDELINES FOR USE:** Take carotenoid supplements with foods that contain a little fat, which allows the body to absorb them more effectively. If you divide in half the total daily amount of supplements you plan to take, and take each half at a different time, your body may be able to absorb more of them.

Possible side effects

Large doses of carotenoids, consumed in food or in the form of supplements, can turn your skin orange, especially the palms of your hands and the soles of your feet. This effect is harmless and will gradually go away if you reduce your intake. Although there are no other known side effects associated with large amounts of mixed carotenoids, taking high doses of particular carotenoids may interfere with the workings of the other carotenoids. Beta-carotene supplements, on their own, do not appear to reduce the risk of any disease, and may increase risk in smokers and those at high risk of lung cancer.

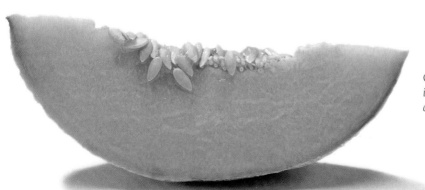

Cantaloupe melon is a good source of beta-carotene.

Cat's claw

Uncaria tomentosa
U. guianensis

First used in European medicine as recently as the 1980s, cat's claw has long been popular among South American Indians as a treatment for wounds, stomach disorders, arthritis, cancer and other ailments. It is a herb derived from the bark or roots of an Amazonian vine.

Common uses

- *May enhance immunity, which makes it useful for sinusitis and other infections.*
- *Supports cancer treatment.*
- *May help to relieve chronic pain.*
- *Reduces pain and inflammation from gout or arthritis.*

Forms

- Capsule
- Dried herb/tea
- Softgel
- Tablet
- Tincture

CAUTION!

- **Do not take cat's claw if you are pregnant, considering pregnancy or breastfeeding. Its safety is not established in these situations, and it may bring on a spontaneous miscarriage.**

REMINDER: If you have a medical condition, consult your doctor before taking supplements.

What it is

In the Amazon basin, one woody tropical vine twining up trees in the rain forest has two curved thorns that resemble the claws of a cat at the base of its leaves. The herb derived from the inner bark or the roots of this plant is known as cat's claw or, in Spanish, *uña de gato*. Although there are dozens of related species, two specific ones, *Uncaria tomentosa* and U. *guianensis*, are harvested in the wild (primarily in Peru and Brazil) for medicinal purposes. Large pieces of their bark are a common sight in South American farmers' markets.

What it does

Modern scientific studies have identified several active ingredients in cat's claw that enhance the activity of the immune system and inhibit inflammation. Their presence may help to explain why this herb has traditionally been used to fight cancer, arthritis, dysentery, ulcers and other infectious and inflammatory conditions. However, there is a lack of clinical evidence to confirm these uses.

MAJOR BENEFITS: Doctors in Germany and Austria prescribe cat's claw to stimulate the immune response in cancer patients who may be weakened by chemotherapy, radiotherapy or other conventional treatments. Several compounds in the herb – some of which have been studied for decades – may account for its cancer-fighting and immunity-boosting effects. In the 1970s researchers reported that the inner bark and root contained compounds called procyanidolic oligomers (PCOs), which inhibit the growth of tumours in animals, and in the 1980s German scientists identified other compounds in cat's claw that enhance the immune system, in part by stimulating immune cells called phagocytes that engulf and devour viruses, bacteria and other disease-causing

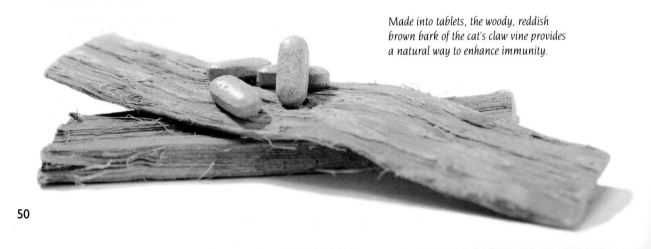

Made into tablets, the woody, reddish brown bark of the cat's claw vine provides a natural way to enhance immunity.

microorganisms. Then in 1993 an Italian study detected another class of compound, quinovic acid glycosides, which have multiple benefits; they act as antioxidants, ridding the body of cell-damaging molecules called free radicals and also kill viruses, reduce inflammation and inhibit the transformation of normal cells into cancerous ones.

In addition to its potential for impeding the growth of tumours, cat's claw may also combat stubborn infections such as sinusitis.

✴ **ADDITIONAL BENEFITS:** Traditionally cat's claw has been relied on to treat pain. Its anti-inflammatory properties apparently make it effective in relieving joint pain caused by arthritis or gout. Additional research is needed, however, to define the precise role that the herb plays in treating arthritis and other inflammatory complaints.

Preliminary reports found that, when used in conjunction with conventional AIDS drugs, cat's claw may benefit people infected with HIV, because it seems to boost the immune response. Some researchers caution against taking the herb for chronic conditions affecting the immune system, including tuberculosis, multiple sclerosis and rheumatoid arthritis, because they believe it may overstimulate the immune system and make symptoms worse. There are doctors, however, who recommend it for autoimmune disorders, including rheumatoid arthritis and lupus. Further studies are required.

How to take it

🖉 **DOSAGE:** Take 250 mg of a standardised extract in tablet form twice a day. Alternatively, take 1 to 2 ml (20 to 40 drops) of the tincture twice a day. The crude herb (the ground root or inner bark of cat's claw in a non-concentrated form) is available in the form of 500 or 1000 mg capsules; these should be taken twice daily (up to 2000 mg a day). Cat's claw tea is sold in health-food shops; use 1 or 2 teaspoons of dried herb per cup of very hot water, following the instructions on the packet. You can drink up to three cups a day.

◉ **GUIDELINES FOR USE:** You can combine or rotate cat's claw with other herbs that stimulate the immune system, such as echinacea, goldenseal, reishi and maitake mushrooms, astragalus and pau d'arco.

Pregnant or breastfeeding women should avoid cat's claw. In Peru it has been valued for a long time as a contraceptive; in animals it stimulates uterine contractions. This effect suggests that the herb could induce miscarriages. It should not be used as a contraceptive.

Possible side effects

Although few studies have been conducted into the safety of cat's claw, there have been no reports that it is toxic at recommended doses. Taking higher doses, however, may cause diarrhoea.

Cayenne and chilli

Hot peppers renowned for the fiery taste they bring to Indian, Mexican and other cuisines, cayenne and chilli are also used medicinally to stimulate digestion and to relieve pain. Their healing properties come from oily compounds called capsaicinoids.

Capsicum genus

Common uses

Topical ointment

- *Alleviates arthritis pain.*

- *Reduces nerve pain associated with shingles (post-herpetic neuralgia), diabetes, surgery or trigeminal neuralgia (tic douloureux).*

Capsule, tablet and tincture

- *Relieve indigestion.*

Forms

- Capsule
- Fresh or dried herb
- Ointment/paste
- Tablet
- Tincture/liquid

What they are

Derived from several varieties of capsicum, cayenne and chilli are cousins of the red and green peppers used in salads and stir-fry dishes, but they are not related to black table pepper. The main active ingredients in the peppers – and what gives them their hotness – are capsaicinoids, particularly capsaicin (pronounced cap-SAY-i-sin), oily irritants that are also the principal ingredients of pepper sprays used in self-defence. Capsaicin is usually described on medicinal labels as 'capsicum'.

What they do

When applied to the skin, capsicum is an effective painkiller. It causes the depletion of a component in nerve cells called substance P, which transmits pain impulses to the brain. When taken as a supplement or in food, capsicum appears to have a highly beneficial effect on the digestive system, and it is sometimes used to counteract poor circulation.

✷ **MAJOR BENEFITS:** Regular application to the skin of an ointment, or paste, containing capsicum can be very effective in relieving arthritis pain. It can also relieve lingering pain in people recovering from shingles, postoperative pain, and pain from nerve damage caused by diabetes.

Preliminary studies indicate that chilli ointment has other medicinal uses. It may reduce the itching of psoriasis (the itching sensation follows the same nerve pathways as pain). The ointment has also shown promise in relieving the aches and pains of fibromyalgia and the coldness in the extremities caused by Raynaud's disease.

✷ **ADDITIONAL BENEFITS:** Fresh peppers, tinctures, tablets and capsules are said to stimulate digestion and to relieve flatulence and ulcers by increasing blood circulation in the stomach and bowel and by promoting the secretion of digestive juices. Liquid products containing tinctures of capsicum can ease symptoms of colds and flu. Claims that capsicum may reduce heart disease risk – by lowering blood cholesterol and triglyceride levels – or help to prevent cancer lack the support of clinical evidence.

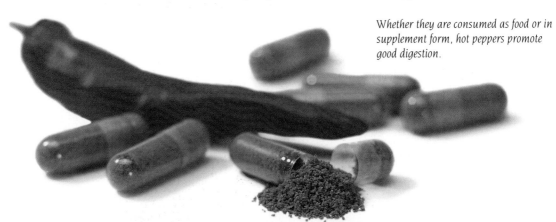

Whether they are consumed as food or in supplement form, hot peppers promote good digestion.

How to take them

⌧ **DOSAGE:** *For external use*: Chilli ointment containing 0.025% to 0.075% capsaicin is most effective with regular, daily use; apply it thinly over the affected areas at least three or four times a day for pain, rubbing it in well. The pain may take several weeks to subside. *Cayenne for internal use*: Follow the instructions on the packet or on the jar of tablets.

◉ **GUIDELINES FOR USE:** *For external use*: Sensitivity to chilli varies from person to person, so test the ointment first on a small, particularly painful area. If it proves effective – which may take a week or more – and causes no lasting discomfort, you can enlarge the coverage area. To avoid getting chilli in the eyes, wash your hands afterwards with warm, soapy water, or wear rubber gloves during application and then discard them; you can also cover the area with a loose bandage. (If you are using chilli ointment to relieve pain in the fingers or hands, wait 30 minutes before washing it off to allow the ointment to penetrate the skin. In the meantime, avoid touching contact lenses and sensitive areas, such as eyes and nose.) Store chilli ointment away from light and extremes of heat or cold, and keep it out of reach of children.

For internal use: Cayenne supplements can be taken with or without food. No adverse effects have been reported in pregnant or breastfeeding women, but discontinue use if a breastfeeding baby becomes irritable.

Possible side effects

Chilli ointment often causes a mildly unpleasant burning sensation that lasts half an hour or so in the first few days of application, but this effect usually disappears after several days of regular use. Using too much ointment or inhaling it may trigger coughing, sneezing, tears or an irritated throat. Chilli can also cause intense pain and burning – though no lasting damage – if it gets in your eyes (or other moist mucous membranes). If this happens, flush the affected area with water or milk. To remove chilli from the skin, wash with warm, soapy water. Vinegar may also work, but do not use it in or near your eyes.

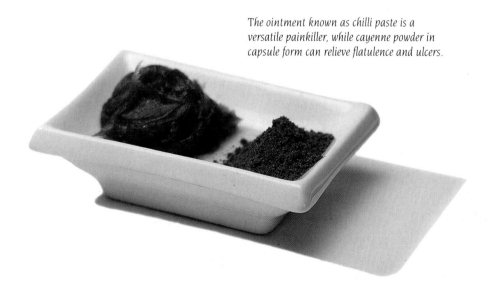

The ointment known as chilli paste is a versatile painkiller, while cayenne powder in capsule form can relieve flatulence and ulcers.

Chamomile

Matricaria recutita

Sometimes called the most soothing plant on earth, chamomile has traditionally been enjoyed as a tea to relax the nerves and ease digestive complaints. The herb is found in concentrated form in pills and tinctures, and in skin formulas designed to treat sores and rashes.

Common uses

- *Promotes general relaxation and relieves anxiety.*
- *Alleviates insomnia.*
- *Heals mouth sores and treats gum disease.*
- *Soothes skin rashes and burns, including sunburn.*
- *Relieves red and irritated eyes.*
- *Eases menstrual cramps.*
- *Treats bowel inflammation, digestive upset and indigestion.*

Forms

- Capsule
- Cream/ointment
- Dried herb/tea
- Oil
- Tincture

CAUTION!

REMINDER: If you have a medical condition, consult your doctor before taking supplements.

What it is

The more popular of the two chamomile herbs (and the one discussed in this book) is German – sometimes called Hungarian – chamomile. It comes from the dried daisy-like flowers of the *Matricaria recutita* plant (its older botanical names are *Matricaria chamomilla* and *Chamomilla recutita*). The other type of chamomile is Roman or English chamomile (*Chamaemelum nobile* or *Anthemis nobilis*), which has properties similar to those of the German species.

The herb has long been used to prepare a gently soothing tea. Its pleasing apple-like aroma and flavour (the name chamomile is derived from the Greek *kamai melon*, meaning 'ground apple') make the ritual of brewing and sipping the tea a relaxing experience in itself.

Concentrated chamomile extracts are added to creams and lotions or packaged as capsules or tinctures. The healing properties of the herb are related in part to its volatile oils, which contain a compound called apigenin as well as other therapeutic substances.

What it does

Chamomile is a great soother. Its anti-inflammatory, antispasmodic and infection-fighting effects can benefit the whole body. When taken internally it calms digestive upsets, relieves cramps and relaxes the nerves. It also works externally on the skin and the mucous membranes of the mouth and eyes, relieving rashes, sores and inflammation.

MAJOR BENEFITS: When Peter Rabbit's mother put him to bed to recover from an adventure, she gave him a spoonful of chamomile tea. Scientists have since confirmed the wisdom of Beatrix Potter's character; studies in animals have shown that chamomile contains substances that act on the same parts of the brain and nervous system as those affected by anti-anxiety drugs, promoting relaxation and reducing stress.

Chamomile appears to have a mildly sedative effect, but more importantly it also calms the body, making it easier for the person taking it to fall asleep naturally. In addition the herb has a relaxing, anti-inflammatory effect on the smooth muscles lining the digestive tract. It helps to relieve a wide range of gastrointestinal complaints, including indigestion, diverticular disorders and inflammatory bowel disease. Its muscle-relaxing action may alleviate menstrual cramps.

ADDITIONAL BENEFITS: Used externally, chamomile helps to soothe skin inflammation. It contains bacteria-fighting compounds that may also speed the healing of infections. A dressing soaked in chamomile tea is often beneficial when applied to mild burns. For sunburn, chamomile oil can be added to a cool bath or mixed with almond oil and rubbed on sunburnt areas. The oil should always be diluted before application, and should never be taken internally. Chamomile creams can also relieve sunburn and skin rashes such as eczema. Alternatively, the herb is used to treat inflammation or infection of the eyes or mouth. Eyewashes made from the cooled tea may relieve the redness or irritation of conjunctivitis and other eye inflammations; prepare a fresh batch of tea daily and store it in a sterile container. Used daily as a gargle or mouthwash, the tea can help to heal mouth sores and prevent gum disease. Inhaled chamomile vapours may also help colds. A study of 60 patients with colds found a better reduction in symptoms with a steam inhalation using chamomile extract, than one using alcohol.

How to take it

☑ **DOSAGE:** *To make a cup of chamomile tea:* Pour a cup of very hot (not boiling) water over 2 teaspoons of dried flowers. Steep for 5 minutes and strain. Drink up to three cups a day or a cup at bedtime. If you are using the tea on the skin or eyes, it should be cooled thoroughly, poured into a sterile container and kept covered until needed. *For the skin:* Add a few drops of chamomile oil to 3 teaspoons of almond oil (or another neutral oil), or buy a ready-made cream. Capsules and tinctures are also available; follow instructions on the packet. A single capsule, or up to 1 teaspoon of tincture, often has the therapeutic effects of a cup of tea.

◉ **GUIDELINES FOR USE:** Chamomile is gentle and can be used over long periods. It can be combined safely with prescription and over-the-counter drugs as well as with other herbs and nutritional supplements. At recommended doses, the herb seems to be safe for children and pregnant and breastfeeding women.

Possible side effects

Whether the herb is used internally or externally, side effects are virtually unknown. Those taking doses higher than recommended of the herb have reported a few instances of nausea and vomiting. Although some concerns have been raised about possible allergic reactions which cause bronchial tightness or skin rashes, these appear to be extremely rare.

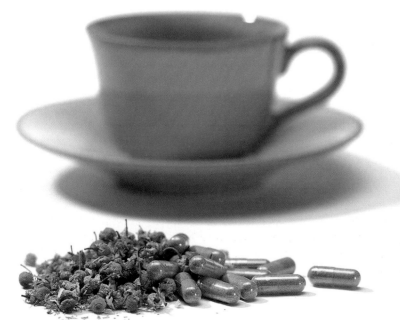

A single capsule can produce the same relaxing effect as a cup of chamomile tea.

Chasteberry

The physicians of ancient Greece, including Hippocrates, recommended chasteberry for the treatment of a variety of conditions. It is now one of the herbs most often prescribed to relieve the symptoms of premenstrual syndrome (PMS) and other menstrual problems.

Vitex agnus-castus

Common uses

- Alleviates symptoms of premenstrual syndrome (PMS).
- Regulates menstruation.
- Promotes fertility.
- Eases menopausal hot flushes.

Forms

- Capsule
- Dried herb/tea
- Tablet
- Tincture

CAUTION!

- Chasteberry affects hormone production, so it should not be used by women taking hormonal medications, including contraceptive pills and oestrogen, or by those who are pregnant.

REMINDER: If you have a medical condition, consult your doctor before taking supplements.

What it is

Also called vitex, chaste tree berry, or monk's pepper, chasteberry is the fruit of the chaste tree. Actually a small shrub with violet flower spikes and long, slender leaves, the chaste tree is native to the Mediterranean region but grows in subtropical climates throughout the world. Its red berries are harvested in the autumn and then dried. They resemble peppercorns in shape, and the taste they impart to a therapeutic cup of tea is distinctively peppery.

What it does

The use of chasteberry for 'female complaints' dates back to Hippocrates in the fourth century BC. Although the herb does not contain hormones, or hormone-like substances, it prompts the pituitary gland (located at the base of the brain) to send a signal to the ovaries to increase production of the female hormone progesterone. Chasteberry also inhibits the excessive production of prolactin, a hormone that primarily regulates breast-milk production but has other less understood actions as well.

⊛ **MAJOR BENEFITS:** Some scientists believe that women who routinely suffer from PMS produce too little progesterone in the last two weeks of their menstrual cycle. This deficiency causes an imbalance in the body's natural oestrogen-progesterone ratio. Chasteberry restores hormonal equilibrium, relieving such PMS-related complaints as irritability, bloating and depression. Studies in Germany indicate that the herb offers at least some relief for PMS symptoms in about 90% of women – and in a third of them the symptoms disappear. Chasteberry's prolactin-lowering action helps to reduce the breast pain and tenderness that some women experience before menstruation even if they have no other premenstrual symptoms.

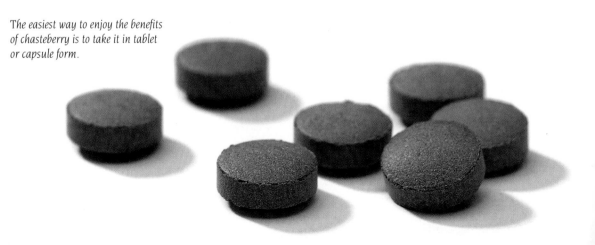

The easiest way to enjoy the benefits of chasteberry is to take it in tablet or capsule form.

✱ **ADDITIONAL BENEFITS:** Because high levels of prolactin and low levels of progesterone in the body can inhibit monthly ovulation, chasteberry may be useful to those who are having trouble becoming pregnant. The herb works best in women with mild or moderately low progesterone levels. When too much prolactin causes menstruation to stop (a condition called amenorrhoea) the herb can help restore a normal monthly cycle.

Menopausal hot flushes are also the result of hormonal changes controlled by the pituitary gland, so women who are experiencing the menopause may want to try chasteberry. Used either alone or in combination with other herbs such as dong quai or black cohosh, it can alleviate the periodic flushing and sweating that occur.

Chasteberry is sometimes also recommended in the treatment of menstrual-related acne.

How to take it

✑ **DOSAGE:** Whether you are using chasteberry to treat PMS, breast tenderness, infertility, amenorrhoea or other menstrual disorders, the dose is the same. In tincture form, add a ½ teaspoon twice a day to a glass of water. The equivalent dose for the powdered extract in tablet or capsule form is 225 mg. For menopausal hot flushes take the same dose (½ teaspoon/225 mg) twice a day.

◉ **GUIDELINES FOR USE:** Take chasteberry on an empty stomach to increase absorption; your first dose should always be taken in the morning. Even after just 10 days a woman with PMS symptoms will probably notice at least some improvement during her next menstrual cycle. However, it may take three months of use to benefit from the full effect of this herb. Six months of treatment with chasteberry may be necessary to correct infertility or amenorrhoea.

Possible side effects

Most people will not notice any adverse side effects from taking chasteberry, but studies have shown that stomach irritation, headache or an itchy rash can occur in a small percentage of women. Discontinue using it if you develop any rash. In addition, some women may experience an increased menstrual flow after taking this herb.

FACTS & TIPS

▪ As with other herbs, the action of chasteberry is the result of the combined effects of several active components; the berry's biological action cannot be reproduced when the components are used individually.

▪ Women who are having trouble breastfeeding may want to try chasteberry, because it can increase milk production. Take 225 mg of chasteberry extract, in tablet or capsule form, twice a day for as long as necessary. The herb does not change the composition of breast milk, so appears safe to use.

Chromium

The trace mineral chromium has been lauded as a slimming aid and a muscle builder as well as a treatment for diabetes and a weapon against heart disease. Although chromium is essential for growth and good health, the more spectacular claims for it remain controversial.

Common uses

- *Essential for the breakdown of protein, fat and carbohydrates.*
- *Helps the body to maintain normal blood sugar (glucose) levels.*
- *May lower total blood cholesterol, LDL ('bad') cholesterol and triglyceride levels.*

Forms

- Capsule
- Liquid
- Softgel
- Tablet

> ### CAUTION!
>
> ■ People with diabetes should consult their doctor before taking chromium. This mineral may alter the dosage for insulin or other diabetes medications.
>
> REMINDER: If you have a medical condition, consult your doctor before taking supplements.

What it is

Chromium is a trace mineral that comes in several chemical forms. As many people do not have enough chromium in their diets, supplements may be worth considering.

What it does

Chromium helps the body to use insulin, a hormone that transfers blood sugar (glucose) to the cells, where it is burned as fuel. With enough chromium the body uses insulin efficiently and maintains normal blood sugar levels. Chromium also aids in breaking down protein and fat.

🛡 **PREVENTION:** A sufficient chromium intake may prevent diabetes in people with insulin resistance. This disorder makes the body less sensitive to the effects of insulin, so the pancreas has to produce more and more of it to keep blood sugar (glucose) levels in check. When the pancreas can no longer keep up with the body's demand for extra insulin, type II diabetes develops. Chromium may avert this outcome by allowing the body to use insulin more effectively in the first place. Chromium also helps to break down fats, so it may reduce LDL ('bad') and increase HDL ('good') cholesterol levels, thus lowering the risk of heart disease.

✳ **ADDITIONAL BENEFITS:** Chromium can relieve headaches, irritability and other symptoms of low blood sugar (hypoglycaemia) by preventing blood sugar levels from dropping below normal. In people with diabetes it may help to control blood sugar levels. Chromium may also help to lower lipid levels and reduce the risk of coronary artery disease. The most controversial claims associated with the mineral relate to weight loss and muscle building. Although some studies indicate that large doses of chromium picolinate can assist weight reduction or increase muscle mass, others have found no benefit. At best, when combined with a sensible diet and regular exercise, mineral supplements may offer a very slight advantage to someone who wants to lose weight. More research is needed to establish chromium's role in this regard.

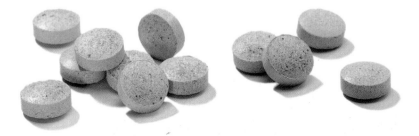

How much you need

No recommended amount has been established for chromium, but scientists believe that 50 to 200 mcg a day can prevent a deficiency in adults. (A daily chromium intake of 200 mcg from food would be hard to achieve even for someone with a healthy, varied diet.)

⊟ **IF YOU GET TOO LITTLE:** A chromium deficiency can lead to inefficient use of glucose. In itself, a lack of chromium is probably not a cause of diabetes, but it can help to bring on the disease in those who are susceptible to it. In addition, anxiety, poor metabolism of amino acids, and high triglyceride and cholesterol levels may occur in individuals who don't get enough chromium.

⊞ **IF YOU GET TOO MUCH:** Chromium supplements do not seem to have any adverse effects even at high doses, although there is some concern that megadoses can impair the absorption of iron and zinc. This can usually be corrected by getting extra iron or zinc through diet or supplements. Supplements containing chromium in the form of chromium picolinate (but not other forms found in supplements) have been linked with cancer and are likely to be banned in the UK.

How to take it

▨ **DOSAGE:** Chromium supplements are generally available in 200 mcg doses. This amount should be taken for general good health, or when following a weight-loss programme or to improve the effectiveness of insulin.

◉ **GUIDELINES FOR USE:** Take chromium in 200 mcg doses with food or a full glass of water to decrease stomach irritation. Chromium is better absorbed when combined with foods high in vitamin C (or taken with a vitamin C supplement). Calcium carbonate supplements or antacids can reduce chromium absorption.

Don't be confused by labels suggesting that one type of chromium – whether picolinate or polynicotinate – is absorbed better than any other. No reliable research supports these claims.

Other sources

Among the foods that contain chromium are whole-grain cereals, potatoes, prunes, peanut butter, nuts, seafood and brewer's yeast. Low-fat diets tend to be higher in chromium than high-fat ones.

DID YOU KNOW?
Whole-grain bread is a good source of chromium. Refined grains, found in white bread, contain little of this essential mineral.

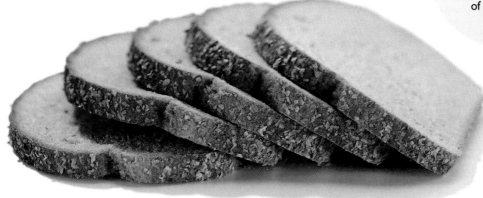

Coenzyme Q$_{10}$

Touted as a wonder supplement, coenzyme Q$_{10}$ is said to enhance stamina, help weight loss, combat cancer and even stave off ageing. These claims are extravagant, but the nutrient does show particular promise in the treatment of heart disease and gum disease.

Common uses

- *Benefits the heart and circulation in cases of heart failure, a weakened heart muscle (cardiomyopathy), high blood pressure, heart rhythm disorders, chest pain (angina) and Raynaud's disease.*

- *Treats gum disease and maintains healthy gums and teeth.*

- *Protects the nerves and may help to slow the progress of Alzheimer's disease and Parkinson's disease.*

- *May help to prevent cancer and heart disease, and may slow down age-related degenerative changes.*

Forms

- Capsule
- Liquid
- Softgel
- Tablet

CAUTION!

■ Pregnant or breastfeeding women should be especially careful about consulting their doctor before using coenzyme Q$_{10}$; the nutrient has not been well studied in this group.

REMINDER: If you have a medical condition, consult your doctor before taking supplements.

What it is

Coenzyme Q$_{10}$, a natural substance produced by the body, belongs to a family of compounds called quinones. When it was first isolated, in 1957, scientists called it ubiquinone because it was ubiquitous in nature. In fact coenzyme Q$_{10}$ is found in all living creatures and is also concentrated in many foods, including nuts and oils. In the past decade coenzyme Q$_{10}$ has become one of the most popular dietary supplements around the world. Proponents of the nutrient use it to maintain general good health as well as to treat heart disease and a number of other serious conditions. Some clinicians believe that it is so important in maintaining the normal functioning of the body that it should be dubbed 'vitamin Q'.

What it does

The primary function of coenzyme Q$_{10}$ is as a catalyst for metabolism – the complex chain of chemical reactions during which food is broken down into packets of energy that the body can use. Acting in conjunction with enzymes (hence the name 'coenzyme') the compound speeds up the metabolic process, providing energy that the cells need to digest food, heal wounds, maintain healthy muscles and perform countless other bodily functions. The nutrient has an essential role in energy production, so it is not surprising that it is found in every cell in the body. Especially abundant in the energy-intensive cells of the heart, it helps this organ to beat more than 100,000 times each day. In addition coenzyme Q$_{10}$ acts as an antioxidant, much like vitamins C and E, helping to neutralise the cell-damaging molecules known as free radicals.

▼ **PREVENTION:** Coenzyme Q$_{10}$ may have a role in preventing cancer, heart attacks and other diseases linked to free-radical damage. It is also

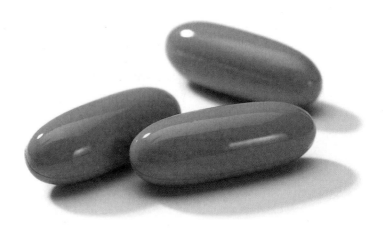

used as an energy enhancer and anti-ageing supplement. Levels of the compound reduce with age (and with certain diseases), so some doctors recommend starting daily supplementation at about the age of 40.

✳ **MAJOR BENEFITS:** Coenzyme Q_{10} has generated much excitement as a possible therapy for heart disease patients, especially those suffering from heart failure or weakened hearts. In some studies patients with poorly functioning hearts improved greatly after adding the supplement to their conventional drugs and therapies. Other studies have shown that people with cardiovascular disease have low levels of this substance in their hearts. Further research suggests that coenzyme Q_{10} may protect against blood clots, reduce blood pressure, diminish irregular heartbeats, treat mitral valve prolapse, lessen symptoms of Raynaud's disease (poor circulation in the extremities) and relieve chest pains (angina). But it is intended as a complement to – not as a replacement for – conventional medical treatments. Do not take this nutrient in place of heart drugs or other prescribed medications.

✳ **ADDITIONAL BENEFITS:** A few small studies suggest that coenzyme Q_{10} may prolong survival in those with breast or prostate cancer, but results remain inconclusive. It also appears to aid healing and reduce pain and bleeding in those with gum disease, and to speed recovery following oral surgery. The supplement shows some promise against Parkinson's and Alzheimer's diseases and fibromyalgia, and it may improve stamina in those with AIDS. Certain practitioners believe that the nutrient helps to stabilise blood sugar levels in people with diabetes.

There are many other claims made for the supplement: that it slows ageing, aids weight loss, enhances athletic performance, combats chronic fatigue syndrome, relieves multiple allergies and boosts immunity. More research is needed to determine the effectiveness of coenzyme Q_{10} for these and other conditions.

How to take it

☑ **DOSAGE:** The general dosage is 50 mg twice a day. Higher dosages of 100 mg twice a day may be useful for heart or circulatory disorders, or for Alzheimer's disease and other specific complaints.

◑ **GUIDELINES FOR USE:** Take a supplement morning and evening, ideally with food to enhance absorption. Coenzyme Q_{10} should be continued over a long period; it may require eight weeks or longer for results to be noticed.

Possible side effects

Most research suggests that the supplement is harmless, even in large doses. In rare cases it may cause upset stomach, diarrhoea, nausea or loss of appetite. As coenzyme Q_{10} has not been extensively studied, however, it is advisable to consult your doctor before using it, especially if you are pregnant or breastfeeding.

Copper

Essential in preventing cardiovascular disease, maintaining good skin and hair colour and promoting fertility, copper is found in at least 15 proteins in the human body. But some nutritionists believe that many people may be marginally deficient in this important nutrient.

Common uses

- *Strengthens blood vessels, bones, tendons and nerves.*
- *Helps to maintain fertility.*
- *Ensures healthy hair and skin pigmentation.*
- *Promotes blood clotting.*

Forms

- **Capsule**
- **Tablet**

CAUTION!

REMINDER: If you have a medical condition, consult your doctor before taking supplements.

What it is

Copper, the reddish brown malleable metal commonly used in cookware and plumbing, is also present as a trace element throughout the human body. This mineral is available in nutritional supplement form as copper carbonate, copper citrate and copper gluconate. Although copper can be obtained from a wide variety of foods, the typical British diet is low in it because the foods that are the best sources, such as shellfish, liver, whole grains, beans, nuts and seeds, are not eaten frequently.

What it does

Copper is essential in the formation of collagen, a fundamental protein in bones, skin and connective tissue. It plays an important role in the development of red blood cells, and may also help the body to use its stored iron and play a role in maintaining immunity and fertility. Involved in the formation of melanin (a dark natural colour found in the hair, skin and eyes), copper also promotes consistent pigmentation.

🛡 **PREVENTION:** Evidence suggests that copper can be a factor in preventing high blood pressure and heart rhythm disorders (arrhythmias). And some researchers believe that it may protect tissues from damage by free radicals, helping to prevent cancer, heart disease and other ailments. Getting enough copper may also help keep to cholesterol levels low.

✳ **ADDITIONAL BENEFITS:** Copper is necessary for the manufacture of many enzymes, especially superoxide dismutase (SOD), which appears to be one of the body's most potent antioxidants. It may also help to stave off bone loss that can lead to osteoporosis.

How much you need

Although there is no daily RDA for copper, adults are advised to obtain 1.5 to 3 mg daily to keep the body functioning normally.

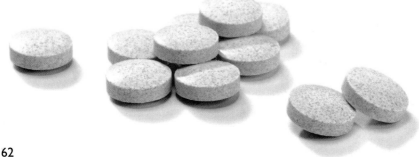

⊟ **IF YOU GET TOO LITTLE:** A true copper deficiency is rare. It usually occurs only in individuals with illnesses such as Crohn's disease or coeliac disease, or in those with inherited conditions that inhibit copper absorption, such as albinism. Symptoms of deficiency are: fatigue; heart rhythm disorders; brittle, discoloured hair; high blood pressure; anaemia; skeletal defects; and infertility.

But even a mild deficiency may have some adverse health effects. For example, a preliminary study involving 24 men found that a diet low in copper caused a significant increase in LDL ('bad') cholesterol and a decrease in HDL ('good') cholesterol. These changes in their cholesterol profiles increased the participants' risk of heart disease.

⊕ **IF YOU GET TOO MUCH:** Just 10 mg of copper taken at one time can produce nausea, muscle pain and stomachache. Severe copper toxicity from oral copper supplements has not been noted to date. However, some people who work with pesticides containing copper have suffered liver damage, coma and even death.

How to take it

☑ **DOSAGE:** Unless a practitioner advises otherwise, copper should only be taken in the form of a multivitamin or multimineral supplement that provides no more than 1 mg of copper daily.

◉ **GUIDELINES FOR USE:** It is advisable to take a supplement at the same time every day, preferably with a meal to decrease the chance of stomach irritation.

Other sources

Shellfish (oysters, lobsters, crabs) and offal are excellent sources of copper. However, if you are concerned about your cholesterol levels, there are many vegetarian foods rich in copper as well. These include legumes; whole grains, such as rye and wheat, and products made from them (bread, cereal, pasta); nuts and seeds; vegetables such as peas, artichokes, avocados, radishes, garlic, mushrooms and potatoes; fruits such as tomatoes, bananas and prunes; and soya products.

RECENT FINDINGS

Copper may help to prevent osteoporosis. In a recent study involving healthy women aged 45 to 56, those taking a daily 3 mg copper supplement showed no loss in bone density, but women given a placebo showed a significant loss.

DID YOU KNOW?

One medium avocado will provide you with about a sixth of the copper that you need each day to maintain optimal health.

Cranberry

Tangy, ruby-red cranberries, often used for making sauce or jelly to accompany roast turkey, have long been considered nature's cure for urinary tract infections, which particularly afflict women of all ages. Modern science has confirmed the merit of this folk wisdom.

Vaccinium macrocarpon

Common uses

- Treats lower urinary tract infections (also called bladder infections or cystitis).
- May prevent recurrence of urinary tract infections.
- Helps to deodorise urine.

Forms

- Capsule
- Fresh or dried fruit
- Juice
- Liquid/tincture
- Powder
- Softgel
- Tablet
- Tea

CAUTION!

- Cranberry is not a substitute for antibiotics in treating an acute urinary tract infection. Consult your doctor if you don't feel better after 24 to 36 hours of using cranberry for a suspected infection.

- Consult your doctor at once if symptoms include fever, shivering, back pain or blood in the urine, which may be signs of a kidney infection requiring medical attention.

REMINDER: *If you have a medical condition, consult your doctor before taking supplements.*

What it is

The cranberry, a native American plant closely related to the blueberry, has been used for centuries in both healing and cooking. The name is a shortened form of craneberry – the flowers of the low-growing shrub were thought to resemble the heads of the cranes that frequented the bogs where it grew. The berries are now widely cultivated throughout the USA. As a traditional medicine, cranberries were crushed and used as poultices for treating wounds and tumours, and also as a remedy for scurvy, a gum and bleeding disorder caused by a deficiency of vitamin C. More recently, medical interest in the cranberry has focused on its role in preventing and treating urinary tract infections (UTIs), which are caused by E. *coli* and other types of bacteria.

What it does

In the 1920s it was discovered that people who consumed large amounts of cranberries produced a more acidic, 'purer' urine. The effect of the cranberries was to stimulate the creation of a powerful substance called hippuric acid, which proved to have a strong antibiotic effect on the urinary tract. It was realised that hippuric acid

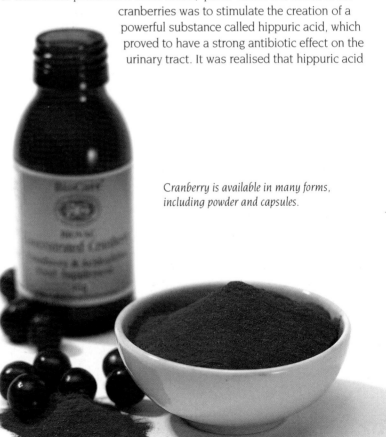

Cranberry is available in many forms, including powder and capsules.

discouraged and sometimes even eliminated infection-causing bacteria. However, more recent studies show that cranberry's main infection-fighting capabilities may be the result of a different property of the fruit. Cranberry appears to inhibit the adhesion of harmful microorganisms to certain cells lining the urinary tract. This makes the environment a less hospitable place for E. *coli* and other disease-causing bacteria to breed, and thereby reduces the likelihood of infection. It is believed that the substances responsible for this effect are a group of phytochemicals known as proanthocyanidins; they are present in cranberry juice but absent from grapefruit, orange, guava, mango and pineapple juices.

MAJOR BENEFITS: Scientists have now confirmed the effectiveness of cranberry in preventing and treating urinary tract infections. Several studies have shown that daily consumption of cranberry, in either juice or capsule form, dramatically reduces the recurrence of such infections. Women are ten times more likely to develop these infections than men – 25% to 35% of women aged 20 to 40 have had at least one – but there is no reason why men should not benefit from cranberry as well.

Cranberry also appears to shorten the course of urinary tract illness, helping to alleviate pain, burning, itching and other symptoms. It is important to remember, though, that persistent urinary tract infections should be treated promptly with antibiotics to prevent complications. However, cranberry juice can be safely taken in combination with conventional drugs. It may even hasten the healing process.

ADDITIONAL BENEFITS: Cranberry helps to deodorise urine, so it should be included in the diet of anyone suffering from the embarrassing odours associated with incontinence. In addition, cranberry's high vitamin C content makes it a natural vitamin supplement. Research also indicates that cranberry may help to reduce cholesterol levels in the blood. A recent US study showed that drinking three glasses of cranberry juice each day significantly raises HDL (good) cholesterol and increases antioxidant levels in the blood, and may reduce the risk of heart disease.

How to take it

DOSAGE: *To treat urinary tract infections*: Take about 800 mg of cranberry extract a day (two 400 mg capsules), or you can drink at least 500 ml of undiluted juice a day or take it in tincture form; follow the instructions on the packet. *To prevent recurrences*: The dose can be halved to 400 mg of cranberry extract a day, or at least 250 ml of juice.

GUIDELINES FOR USE: Cranberry can be taken with or without food. Drinking plenty of water or other fluids in addition to cranberry and throughout the day should speed recovery. Cranberry has no known interactions with antibiotics or other medications, but by acidifying the urine it may lessen the effect of another herb, uva ursi (also known as bearberry), which is sometimes used for urinary tract infections.

Possible side effects

There are no known side effects from either short-term or long-term use of cranberry. It also appears to be safe for consumption by pregnant or breastfeeding women.

Dandelion

Taraxacum officinale

Known mostly as a persistent and prolific weed, dandelion is grown commercially in several countries. Its leaves and roots are a rich source of vitamins and minerals, and its active ingredients are particularly useful for treating digestive and liver problems.

Common uses

- *The root strengthens liver function: useful in cases of hepatitis (liver inflammation) and jaundice.*
- *The root aids digestion by stimulating the release of bile from the liver and gallbladder; may help to prevent gallstones.*
- *The root helps to reduce oestrogen dominance in endometriosis and breast pain.*
- *The leaves help to reduce fluid retention.*

Forms

- Capsule
- Dried or fresh herb/tea
- Liquid
- Tablet
- Tincture

CAUTION!

- **Dandelion should not be used during acute attacks of gallstones. Seek medical advice.**

REMINDER: If you have a medical condition, consult your doctor before taking supplements.

What it is

Dandelion grows wild throughout much of the world and is cultivated in parts of Europe for medicinal uses. Closely related to chicory, the plant can grow 30 cm high; its spatula-shaped leaves are shiny, hairless and deeply serrated. The solitary yellow flower blooms for much of the growing season, opening at daybreak and closing at dusk and in wet weather (some cultures have used dandelions to signal the approach of rain). After the flower matures, the plant forms a puffball of seeds that are dispersed by the wind (or by playful children). Supplements usually contain the root (which is tapered and sweet tasting) or leaves, though the whole plant and flowers are also valued for their healing properties.

What it does

Folk healers have long prescribed dandelion root for liver and digestive problems, and the leaf for fluid retention. Dandelion's various active ingredients enhance the performance of the liver and kidneys, so the plant is useful for a wide range of disorders where the elimination of toxins is indicated.

MAJOR BENEFITS: Studies of dandelion's beneficial effects on the liver have shown that the herb increases the production and flow of bile (a digestive aid) from the liver and gallbladder, helping to treat such conditions as gallstones, jaundice and hepatitis. The leaf has a strong diuretic action which has been ascribed to its content of potassium, a natural diuretic. Dandelion is sometimes mixed with other nutritional supplements that reinforce liver function, including milk thistle, black radish, celandine, beet leaf, fringe tree bark, inositol, methionine and choline. Such combinations are usually sold as liver or lipotropic ('fat-metabolising') formulas in health-food shops.

Its capacity to improve liver function means that dandelion root (in combination with other liver-strengthening nutrients) may be effective for relieving the symptoms of oestrogen excess, such as endometriosis and cyclical breast pain. By enhancing the liver's ability to remove excess oestrogen from the body, it helps to restore a healthy balance of hormones in women who are afflicted with these disorders.

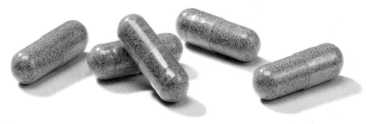

✳ **ADDITIONAL BENEFITS:** Dandelion root acts as a mild laxative, so a tea made from it may provide a gentle remedy for constipation. The herb can also enhance the body's ability to absorb iron from either food or supplements, which makes it useful in some cases of anaemia. Early research suggests that dandelion may be of value in treating cancer: the Japanese have patented a freeze-dried extract of dandelion root to use against tumours, and the Chinese are using dandelion extracts to treat breast cancer (an approach supported by positive effects in animal studies). But additional studies need to be conducted in humans to determine the herb's true effectiveness against specific types of cancer.

Researchers have found that dandelion can lower blood sugar levels in animals, which suggests that it may have a role to play in the treatment of diabetes. The diuretic effect of the leaves makes them a useful treatment for water retention and bloating.

How to take it

✐ **DOSAGE:** *To strengthen liver function in cases of hepatitis, gallstones and endometriosis*: Take 500 mg of a powdered solid dandelion-root extract twice a day. This amount may also be found in some lipotropic (liver) combinations. Or take 1 or 2 teaspoons of a liquid dandelion extract three times a day. *For constipation*: Drink one cup of dandelion root tea three times a day. *For anaemia*: Have 1 teaspoon of fresh dandelion juice or tincture each morning and evening with half a glass of water. *For water retention*: Drink one cup of dandelion leaf tree three times a day.

◎ **GUIDELINES FOR USE:** Drink fresh dandelion juice or liquid extract with water. Capsules and tablets containing dandelion root extract can be consumed with or without food. No adverse effects have been reported in pregnant or breastfeeding women.

Possible side effects

Dandelion has no serious side effects. In large doses it may cause a skin rash, upset stomach or diarrhoea. Stop using it if this happens, and discuss the reaction with your doctor.

FACTS & TIPS

■ To make dandelion tea, use the dried chopped root or leaves of the dandelion. Pour a cup of very hot water over 1 or 2 teaspoons of the herb and allow it to steep for about 15 minutes. The tea can be blended with other herbs, such as liquorice, and sweetened with honey.

■ Dandelion is a health-giving and nutritious food or drink. Both the leaves and the flowers taste good when steamed like spinach, and the pleasantly bitter greens make a tangy addition to salads. Juice can be extracted from the leaves, and the root can be roasted and used to brew a drink that substitutes for coffee (without the stimulant effects).

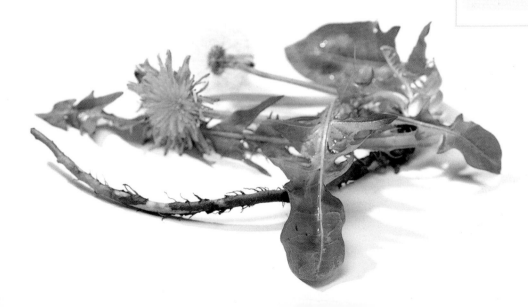

Dong quai

Angelica sinensis
A. acutiloba

An ingredient in many herbal 'women's supplements', dong quai, or Chinese angelica, is a traditional tonic used in Asia to aid the female reproductive system. Its popularity is second only to ginseng's in China and Japan, but Western experts continue to debate the effectiveness of this herb.

Common uses

- *May help to ease menstrual cramps.*
- *May reduce hot flushes associated with the menopause.*

Forms

- Capsule
- Dried herb/tea
- Liquid
- Softgel
- Tablet
- Tincture

CAUTION!

- Dong quai should not be used by pregnant women or those who are breastfeeding.

- People on anticoagulant drugs should seek medical advice before taking dong quai.

- Dong quai may exacerbate heavy menstrual bleeding and increase the skin's sensitivity to the sun.

REMINDER: If you have a medical condition, consult your doctor before taking supplements.

What it is

Although dong quai grows wild in Asia, it is also widely cultivated for medicinal purposes in China (the species Angelica sinensis) and in Japan (A. *acutiloba*), where many women take it daily to maintain overall good health. The most widely available therapeutic form is derived from the root of A. *sinensis*, a plant with hollow stems that grows up to 2.5 m tall and has clusters of white flowers. When in bloom, angelica resembles Queen Anne's lace, its botanical relative. Other names for dong quai include dang gui, tang kuie and Chinese angelica.

What it does

Dong quai is believed to keep the uterus healthy and to regulate the menstrual cycle. It may also widen blood vessels and increase blood flow to various organs. Even among herbal experts, however, questions linger about its benefits. One reason dong quai has been difficult to assess is that it is often taken in combination with other herbs.

✪ **MAJOR BENEFITS:** Traditionally, dong quai has been used in the treatment of menstrual and menopausal problems. The herb has been claimed to correct abnormal bleeding patterns, to alleviate symptoms of premenstrual syndrome (PMS), to ease menstrual cramps, to reduce menopausal hot flushes and to lessen the vaginal dryness associated with the menopause.

There are two theories about how dong quai helps to combat these ailments. Some herbalists believe that it contains plant oestrogens (phytoestrogens), which are weaker than oestrogens produced by the body but which form chemical bonds with oestrogen receptors in human cells. Phytoestrogens are effective in restoring hormonal equilibrium; for example, they can prevent hot flushes by compensating for the decline in oestrogen levels that occurs after the menopause.

Other researchers attribute the effectiveness of dong quai to its abundance of coumarins. This group of natural chemicals dilates blood

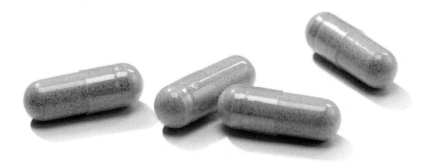

vessels, increases blood flow to the uterus and other organs, and stimulates the central nervous system. Coumarins also appear to reduce inflammation and muscle spasms, which may account for dong quai's ability to reduce the severity of menstrual cramps.

ADDITIONAL BENEFITS: Although dong quai is not typically used to lower blood pressure, it does have this effect because it dilates blood vessels, making it easier for the heart to pump blood through the body. This has the additional benefit of improving peripheral circulation.

How to take it

DOSAGE: *For PMS, menstrual irregularities, menstrual cramps or hot flushes:* Take 600 mg of dong quai extract daily. The same effect can be obtained from taking 30 drops of tincture three times a day. In capsule, tablet or liquid form, extracts should be standardised to contain 0.8% to 1.1% ligustilide. Alternatively you can also use a preparation in which dong quai is combined with such menstrual-regulating herbs as chasteberry, liquorice and Siberian ginseng.

GUIDELINES FOR USE: For symptoms of PMS, use dong quai on the days when you are not menstruating. If you also suffer from menstrual cramps, continue using dong quai until menstruation stops. For cramps without PMS, begin taking dong quai the day before your period is due. For hot flushes, use it daily. Continue the herb for two months before deciding whether it has achieved the desired effect.

Possible side effects

Dong quai may have a mild laxative effect and may cause heavy menstrual bleeding. Protect yourself from the sun when using dong quai, because its root contains compounds called psoralens that can make some people more sensitive to sunlight and cause severe sunburn.

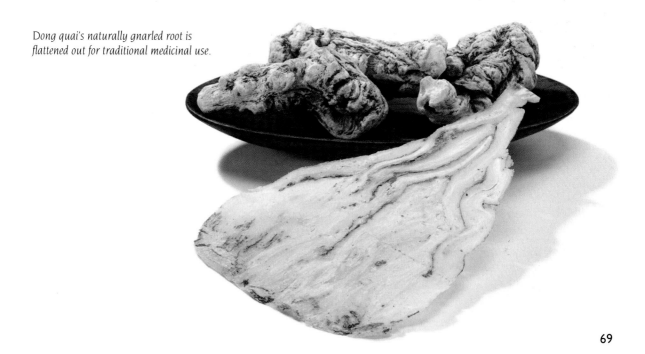

Dong quai's naturally gnarled root is flattened out for traditional medicinal use.

Echinacea

Echinacea angustifolia
E. pallida
E. purpurea

Common uses

- *Reduces the body's susceptibility to colds and flu.*
- *Limits the duration and severity of infections.*
- *Helps to fight thrush and recurrent respiratory, middle-ear and urinary tract infections.*
- *Speeds the healing of skin wounds and inflammations.*

Forms

- Capsule
- Dried herb/tea
- Liquid
- Lozenge
- Softgel
- Tablet
- Tincture

CAUTION!

- If you are taking antibiotics or other drugs for an infection, use echinacea in addition to, rather than as a replacement for, those medications.

- In progressive infections such as tuberculosis, echinacea may not be effective.

REMINDER: *If you have a medical condition, consult your doctor before taking supplements.*

A plant native to the USA, long used by traditional healers and earlier generations of doctors, echinacea fell out of favour with the advent of modern antibiotics. But it is regaining popularity as a safe and powerful immune-system booster to fight colds, flu and other infections.

What it is

Also known as the purple, or prairie, coneflower, echinacea (pronounced ek-in-NAY-sha) is a wild flower with daisy-like purple blossoms, native to the grasslands of the central USA. For centuries the Plains tribes used the plant to heal wounds and to counteract the toxins of snakebites. The herb also became a favourite among European pioneers in America and their doctors as an all-purpose fighter of infections. It is popularly grown in the UK as a garden plant.

Of the nine echinacea species, three (*Echinacea angustifolia*, E. *pallida* and E. *purpurea*) are used medicinally. They appear in literally hundreds of commercial preparations, which utilise different parts of the plant (flowers, leaves, stems or roots) and come in a variety of forms. Echinacea contains many active ingredients thought to strengthen the immune system, and in recent years it has become one of the most extensively used herbal remedies in the world.

What it does

A natural antibiotic and infection fighter, echinacea helps to kill bacteria, viruses, fungi and other disease-causing microbes. It acts by stimulating various immune-system cells that are key weapons against infection. In addition, the herb boosts the cells' production of an innate virus-fighting substance called interferon. These effects are relatively shortlived, however, so it is advisable to take the herb at frequent intervals – as often as every couple of hours during acute infections. Echinacea normalises immune response even in autoimmune conditions such as eczema (for which it is a traditional treatment).

PREVENTION: Echinacea can help to prevent the two most common viral ailments – colds and flu. It is most effective when taken at the first hint of illness. In one study of people who were susceptible to colds, those who used the herb for eight weeks were 35% less likely to come down with a cold than those given a placebo. Furthermore, they caught colds less often – 40 days elapsed between infections, versus 25 days for the placebo group. Studies confirm that echinacea is also useful if you are already suffering from the aches, pains, congestion or fever of colds or flu. Overall, symptoms are less severe and subside sooner.

ADDITIONAL BENEFITS: Echinacea may be of value for recurrent ailments, including thrush and infections of the urinary tract or middle ear. It is also sometimes used to treat streptococcal and staphylococcal infections, herpes infections (including genital herpes, cold sores and shingles), bronchitis and sinus infections. Autoimmune conditions which may respond to echinacea include lupus, multiple sclerosis, rheumatoid arthritis and similar disorders. The herb is also being studied as a treatment for chronic fatigue syndrome and AIDS, and it may prove effective against some types of cancer, particularly in patients whose immune systems have been depressed by radiotherapy or chemotherapy.

Echinacea can be applied to the skin. Its juice promotes the healing of all kinds of wounds, boils, abscesses, eczema, burns, mouth ulcers or cold sores, and bedsores. To treat a sore throat or tonsillitis, the tincture can be diluted and used as a gargle.

How to take it

⊘ **DOSAGE:** Because echinacea comes in many different forms, check the product's label for the proper dosage; most tablets are of powdered root rather than extract. *For colds and flu*: A high dose is needed – up to 200 mg five a times a day. In one major study, patients with flu who were given 900 mg of echinacea a day did better than those who received either a lower dosage of 450 mg a day or a placebo. *For other infections*: The recommended dose is 200 mg three or four times a day. *For long-term use as a general immune booster*: To derive the most benefits, especially for those prone to chronic infections, alternate echinacea every three weeks with other herbs that enhance the immune system, including goldenseal, astragalus, pau d'arco and medicinal mushrooms. Echinacea teas, often blended with other herbs, are available as well.

◉ **GUIDELINES FOR USE:** It is sometimes advised that echinacea should be used for no longer than eight weeks, followed by a one-week interval before you resume taking it. However, medical herbalists often use the herb continuously for the treatment of autoimmune conditions such as eczema. You can take it with or without food.

Possible side effects

At recommended doses, echinacea has no known side effects, and no adverse reactions have been reported in pregnant or breastfeeding women. However, people who are allergic to flowers in the daisy family may also be allergic to this herb. If you develop a skin rash or have trouble breathing, consult your doctor straightaway.

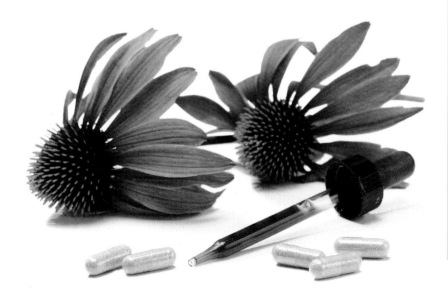

Evening primrose oil

Native Americans introduced the early settlers to the healing powers of the evening primrose. Modern research focuses on the therapeutic effect of the oil from its seeds, which contain a special fatty acid called gamma-linolenic acid (GLA).

Oenothera biennis

Common uses

- *Eases rheumatoid arthritis pain.*
- *Can minimise symptoms of diabetic nerve damage.*
- *Relieves eczema symptoms.*
- *Helps to treat premenstrual syndrome (PMS), endometriosis and menstrual cramps.*
- *Lessens inflammation of acne, rosacea and muscle strains.*

Forms

- Capsule
- Oil
- Softgel

CAUTION!

- People with a history of epilepsy should consult their doctor before taking evening primrose oil. Some reports indicate that high doses may precipitate an attack.

REMINDER: If you have a medical condition, consult your doctor before taking supplements.

What it is

Called evening primrose because its light yellow flowers open at dusk, this wild flower is native to North America. The plant and its root have long been used for medicinal purposes – to treat bruises, haemorrhoids, sore throats and stomach aches – but the use of its seed oil, which contains gamma-linolenic acid (GLA), is relatively recent. GLA is an essential fatty acid that the body converts to hormone-like compounds called prostaglandins, which regulate a number of bodily functions.

Although the body can make GLA from other types of fat, there is no one food that has appreciable amounts of GLA. Evening primrose oil provides a concentrated source: 7% to 10% of its fatty acids are in the form of GLA. But there are other sources of GLA. Borage seed oil and blackcurrant seed oil contain larger quantities of GLA – 20% to 26% for borage; 14% to 19% for blackcurrant – than evening primrose oil, but they also have higher percentages of other fatty acids that may interfere with GLA absorption. Most of the studies investigating the effects of GLA have used evening primrose oil, and for this reason it is the preferred source of GLA. Borage oil may nevertheless be a good substitute: it is cheaper than evening primrose oil, and a lower dose is required to produce a therapeutic effect.

What it does

The body produces several types of prostaglandin; some promote inflammation, others control it. The GLA in evening primrose oil is directly converted to important anti-inflammatory prostaglandins, which accounts for most of the supplement's therapeutic effects. In addition, GLA is an important component of cell membranes.

PREVENTION: The GLA in evening primrose oil appears to inhibit the development of diabetic neuropathy, the nerve damage that is a common complication of diabetes. In a study of people with a mild form of the condition, one year of treatment with evening primrose oil reduced numbness and tingling, loss of sensation and other symptoms of the disorder better than a placebo did, suggesting that evening primrose may be effective in reversing neuropathy.

ADDITIONAL BENEFITS: One of the leading uses for evening primrose oil is to treat eczema, an allergic skin condition that may develop if the body has trouble converting fats from food into GLA. Some studies of people with eczema have indicated that taking evening primrose oil for three to four months can alleviate itching and reduce the need for topical steroid creams and drugs with unpleasant side effects.

Some studies have indicated that evening primrose oil can be effective in treating menstrual disorders such as PMS, menstrual cramps and endometriosis. In particular, the oil blocks the inflammatory prostaglandins that cause menstrual cramps. It also appears to ease the breast tenderness that some women experience just before their periods, and may play a role in reversing infertility in some women.

Rheumatoid arthritis is characterised by joint pain and swelling, and studies have found that these symptoms improve with supplements of evening primrose oil or another source of GLA. Conditions that involve inflammation, such as rosacea, acne and muscle strain, may also benefit from evening primrose oil.

How to take it

⊘ **DOSAGE:** The recommended therapeutic dose for evening primrose oil is generally 1000 mg three times a day. This supplies 240 mg of GLA a day. To get an equivalent amount of GLA from other sources you would need to take 1000 mg of borage oil or 1500 mg of blackcurrant oil each day. Evening primrose oil or borage oil can also be applied topically to the fingers to ease the symptoms of Raynaud's disease.

◉ **GUIDELINES FOR USE:** Take evening primrose oil or other sources of GLA with meals to enhance absorption.

Possible side effects

In studies, about 2% of the participants using evening primrose oil experienced bloating or abdominal upset. However, consuming it with food may lessen this effect.

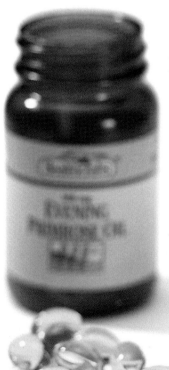

Although evening primrose oil is available as a liquid, it may be more convenient to take it in softgel form.

RECENT FINDINGS

In a study of 60 people with eczema, GLA – the essential fatty acid in evening primrose oil – was found to be superior to a placebo in reducing the itching and oozing of the condition. Those in the GLA group took 274 mg twice a day (an amount found in approximately seven 1000 mg evening primrose capsules) for 12 weeks. Examinations by a dermatologist every four weeks confirmed the gradual improvement of symptoms reported by these patients.

A study from the University of Massachusetts Medical Center showed that very high doses of GLA in the form of borage oil (2.4 grams of GLA a day) reduced damage to joint tissue in people with rheumatoid arthritis. As a result they had less joint pain and swelling.

Feverfew

Tanacetum parthenium

Common uses

■ *Helps to prevent or reduce the intensity of migraines.*

■ *May ease menstrual complaints.*

Forms

■ Capsule
■ Dried herb/tea
■ Tablet
■ Tincture

CAUTION!

■ Pregnant women should avoid feverfew because it may cause contractions of the uterus. Women who are breastfeeding should not use the herb.

■ Feverfew may inhibit blood clotting, so consult your doctor before using it if you are taking anticoagulant drugs.

REMINDER: If you have a medical condition, consult your doctor before taking supplements.

In the Middle Ages feverfew was believed to purify the air and prevent malaria and other life-threatening diseases. It has since been relied on to treat headaches, stomach problems and menstrual irregularities. Most recently the herb has been hailed as a migraine preventative.

What it is

Feverfew – also known as featherfew or febrifuge – is a member of the botanical family that includes daisies and sunflowers. With its bright yellow-and-white blossoms and feathery yellow-green leaves, the herb resembles chamomile and is often mistaken for it. The leaves are used medicinally, and although the flowers have no health benefits they emit a strong aroma. The odour of feverfew is apparently offensive to insects, so if you plant the herb in your garden it will act as a natural repellent.

What it does

The active compound in feverfew, called parthenolide, seems to block substances in the body that widen and constrict blood vessels and cause inflammation.

PREVENTION: Although the exact cause of migraines is unknown, some doctors think that these headaches occur when blood vessels in the head constrict and then rapidly dilate. Such a dramatic change can trigger the release of chemicals that cause pain and inflammation which are stored in platelets (the small blood cells involved in blood clotting). Researchers speculate that feverfew prevents the sudden dilation of blood vessels, and thereby inhibits the release of those chemicals. Although this action makes feverfew a good migraine preventative, the herb cannot relieve a migraine once it occurs.

Word of mouth among people with chronic migraines led to widespread use of feverfew beginning in the 1970s. To determine the

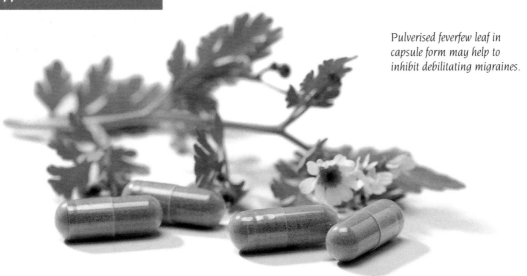

Pulverised feverfew leaf in capsule form may help to inhibit debilitating migraines.

effectiveness of the herb British researchers recruited migraine sufferers who had already been using feverfew regularly. The researchers divided the subjects into two groups: one group continued to take feverfew; the other was given a placebo. Those taking the placebo pills soon experienced more frequent and more intense headaches, but those in the feverfew group had no increase in migraine occurrences. Another study showed that feverfew reduced the number of migraines by 24%, and that, even when the headaches did occur, they were much less severe. The results of these and other studies have led health authorities in Canada and other countries to approve the use of feverfew for migraine prevention.

✳ **ADDITIONAL BENEFITS:** Feverfew has long been used to treat menstrual complaints, in particular menstrual cramps, which result from an excess of prostaglandins produced by the lining of the uterus. Prostaglandins are hormone-like substances that can cause pain and inflammation. Feverfew inhibits the production of them.

The anti-inflammatory action of the herb also encouraged its use as a treatment for the inflamed, sore joints that occur in rheumatoid arthritis. However, a study of arthritis patients found no additional benefit from taking feverfew in conjunction with medications commonly prescribed for the condition. No studies have been done to establish how the herb might work when taken on its own, or in combination with other herbal treatments for rheumatoid arthritis.

How to take it

▨ **DOSAGE:** For migraines, a dose of 250 mg a day of a feverfew product standardised to contain at least 0.4% parthenolide is typical.

◉ **GUIDELINES FOR USE:** The experience of the migraine sufferers in the British study cited above underlines the importance of taking feverfew daily over a long period. If you stop taking the herb after a short time, the headaches may resume.

Possible side effects

Few side effects have been noted, even when feverfew is used long term. There have been reports of sores and inflammation of the mucous membranes of the mouth, but this reaction seems to be limited to people who chew the fresh leaves (a common practice before feverfew supplements became available). Some people experience stomach upsets from both the fresh leaves and supplements. Skin contact with the plant can cause a rash; anyone who develops a rash after touching feverfew should not use the product internally.

BUYING GUIDE

■ One study in the UK reported that half of the feverfew preparations examined contained virtually none of its active ingredient, parthenolide. Look for feverfew tablets and capsules made from the herb *Tanacetum parthenium* and standardised to contain at least 0.4% parthenolide.

CASE HISTORY

A migraine preventative

For a while Nick L. put all his faith in the new migraine drugs because of their amazing ability to stop the dizzying pain of his headaches. But what he really wanted was something that could prevent a migraine from starting. His doctor suggested other drugs, but their side effects were troublesome. 'The beta-blockers saw off my migraines,' Nick remembers, 'but my sex life vanished too.' He tried several types, but the result was always the same.

During a trip to Manchester he saw a shop sign: 'Migraine Sufferers – We have feverfew in stock.' Although he was sceptical of herbal therapies he bought a bottle, which sat unopened in his medicine chest for six months.

Then he read an article affirming the safety and effectiveness of feverfew. He decided to give it a try and took two capsules with his daily vitamin supplement. 'From that point on it was a migraine-free year,' he says, 'my first since childhood.'

Fibre

Hippocrates praised wholemeal bread 'for its salutary effect upon the bowel' but only in the past 30 years has the health significance of fibre been fully recognised. The shift began after two British doctors working in Africa realised that a high-fibre diet could counteract certain Western diseases.

Common uses

- Promotes good digestion and healthy bowels.
- Lowers blood cholesterol.
- Can relieve constipation, diarrhoea, irritable bowel syndrome and haemorrhoid pain.
- Stabilises blood glucose levels.
- Can facilitate weight loss.
- May help to prevent gallstones.

Forms

- Bran-rich cereals
- Granules
- Powder

CAUTION!

- High intakes of fibre can reduce the effectiveness of some drugs, including oral contraceptives and the anti-cholesterol drug lovastatin.

- Swallowing fibre tablets or capsules can be dangerous. When they become hydrated they can expand and create an obstruction in the throat or further down the intestine.

- If you have a rare allergic reaction to psyllium, such as a rash or breathing difficulties, seek immediate medical help.

REMINDER: If you have a medical condition, consult your doctor before taking supplements.

What it is

Fibre provides almost no nutritional value, but soluble and insoluble fibre play an important role in maintaining good health. Soluble fibre – found in fruit, vegetables, oats, nuts and pulses – is made up of gums and other constituents of plant cells and plant cell walls that swell in water. It is broken down into simpler components by the action of bacteria in the large intestine. Psyllium seeds are a commonly used source of soluble fibre. Insoluble fibre – found in grains – consists mainly of the cellulosic constituents of plant cell walls, which bind with water but do not swell appreciably. It passes undigested through the intestines because it cannot be absorbed or broken down by the body's own enzymes.

What it does

Fibre absorbs excess water from the intestine to make larger, softer stools. It also binds to cholesterol which is then expelled, and so is useful for reducing cholesterol levels in the bloodstream. Insoluble fibre, such as cellulose, assists the function of the gut as well as binding with cancer-causing substances and toxins and aiding their excretion. Although soluble fibre cannot be digested, it is fermented by friendly bacteria in the gut, producing fatty acids that are important for nourishing the cells of the intestine.

⬢ MAJOR BENEFITS: A shortage of fibre in the diet has been linked to a number of degenerative, chronic diseases including heart disease, diverticular disorders and diabetes. Although a healthy diet should contain 18 grams of fibre a day, most people in the UK have an average intake of only 12 grams. Eating just one slice of wholemeal bread provides an extra 5 grams of fibre.

A fibre-rich diet can help to prevent constipation and haemorrhoids by increasing the water content of stools, making it easier for them to be passed out of the body. A diet high in soluble fibre can help to reduce the body's need for insulin and assist diabetics by slowing down the absorption of blood sugar. Soluble fibre also reduces the removal of cholesterol from the gut into the bloodstream, leading to lower levels of blood cholesterol. In one study people with high levels of cholesterol were given a minimum of 10 grams of psyllium daily for six weeks or longer. They showed a significantly higher reduction (between 6 and 20%) of LDL ('bad') cholesterol than those on a low-fat diet.

Being a rich source of soluble fibre, psyllium helps to regulate bowel function in people suffering from diarrhoea, as well as constipation. Hence it may be helpful to those with irritable bowel syndrome, where the symptoms can alternate between these extremes.

✴ **ADDITIONAL BENEFITS:** In some studies, fibre has been shown to help weight loss by filling the stomach with absorbed water and decreasing appetite as well as delaying the moment when food leaves the stomach. High-fibre foods, especially linseed, contain plant oestrogens known as lignans which have been linked to a reduced risk of cancer, and of breast cancer in particular. Psyllium may have a role to play in preventing gallstones; a Mexican study of obese patients with an increased risk of gallstones found that psyllium helped to avert the condition.

How to take it

☑ **DOSAGE:** Start with a small dose of between 1 and 2 grams with each meal. This can be increased gradually to between 1 and 3 tablespoons (up to 10 grams) of powder two or three times a day with 250 ml of juice or water. Never take more than 30 grams in one day.

◉ **GUIDELINES FOR USE:** If you are taking fibre supplements ensure that you also have a high intake of liquids because fibre absorbs large quantities of water. After taking fibre supplements it it advisable to wait two hours before taking any medication because the supplements may delay their absorption. Pregnant women should seek medical advice before taking fibre supplements.

Possible side effects

A sudden high intake of fibre may create bloating and abdominal pain. Beans and pulses in particular can cause wind and flatulence. Some people develop gastric irritation when they consume fibre, especially wheat.

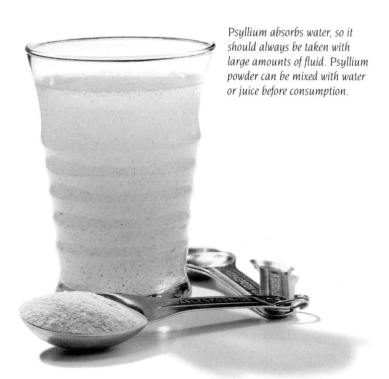

Psyllium absorbs water, so it should always be taken with large amounts of fluid. Psyllium powder can be mixed with water or juice before consumption.

Fish oils

Scientists noticed a curiously low incidence of heart disease among Greenland's Inuits despite their high-fat diet. The reason? They were eating fish rich in omega-3 fatty acids. Later studies confirmed the cardio-protective effect of fish oils while uncovering other benefits as well.

Common uses

- *Help to prevent cardiovascular disease; useful for other circulatory conditions, including lowering levels of triglycerides (blood fats).*

- *Block disease-related inflammatory responses in the body.*

- *May lower blood pressure.*

Forms

- Capsule
- Liquid
- Powder
- Softgel

CAUTION!

- Omega-3 fatty acids inhibit blood clotting, so consult a doctor before using fish oil supplements if you have a blood disorder or if you are taking anticoagulant medications.

- Fish oil supplements should not be taken during the two days before or after surgery.

- People with diabetes should consult their doctors before taking fish oil supplements, as large doses may raise blood sugar levels.

REMINDER: If you have a medical condition, consult your doctor before taking supplements.

What they are

The fat in fish contains a class of polyunsaturated fatty acid called omega-3s. These fatty acids differ from the polyunsaturated fatty acids found in vegetable oils, called omega-6s, and have different effects on the body. (Fish do not manufacture such fats but obtain them from the plankton they eat; the colder the water, the more omega-3s the plankton contains.) The two most potent forms of omega-3s – eicosapentaenoic acid (EPA) and docosahexaenoic acid (DHA) – are found in abundance in cold-water fish such as salmon, trout, mackerel and tuna. The sources of a third type of omega-3, alpha-linolenic acid (ALA), are certain vegetable oils (such as flaxseed oil) and leafy greens (such as purslane). However, ALA may not be as effective as EPA and DHA; this is still being researched.

What they do

Omega-3s play a key role in a range of vital body processes, from regulating blood pressure and blood clotting to boosting immunity. They may be useful for preventing or treating many diseases and disorders.

PREVENTION: Fish oils appear to reduce the risk of heart disease. They do this in several ways. Most importantly, the presence of omega-3s makes platelets in the blood less likely to clump together and form the clots that lead to heart attacks. Next, omega-3s can reduce triglycerides (blood fats carried with cholesterol) and may lower blood pressure. In addition, recent research has shown that omega-3s strengthen the heart's electrical system, preventing heart-rhythm abnormalities. However, the strongest evidence for the cardiovascular benefits of fish oils comes from studies in which the participants ate fish rather than taking fish oil supplements.

Within the artery walls, omega-3s inhibit inflammation, which is a factor in plaque build-up. Therapeutic doses of fish oils are one of the few successful ways to prevent the reblockage of arteries that often occurs after angioplasty (a procedure in which a small balloon is guided through an artery to a blockage and is inflated to compress plaque, widen the vessels and improve blood flow to the heart). This effect on blood vessels makes fish oils helpful for Raynaud's disease as well.

ADDITIONAL BENEFITS: Omega-3s are also effective general anti-inflammatories, useful for joint problems, lupus and psoriasis. Studies indicate that people with rheumatoid arthritis experience less joint swelling and stiffness, and may even be able to manage on lower doses of anti-inflammatory drugs, when they take fish oil supplements. In a study of people with Crohn's disease (a painful type of inflammatory bowel disease), 69% of those taking enteric-coated fish oil supplements (about 3 grams of fish oils a day) experienced no symptoms of their illness, compared with just 28% of those receiving a placebo. Fish oils may also help to ease menstrual cramps. In addition, omega-3s may play a role in mental health: some nutritionists believe that there is a correlation between the increasing incidence of depression in Australia and the declining consumption of fish, and preliminary studies suggest that omega-3 fatty acids may reduce the severity of schizophrenia by about 25%, and also help to correct dyslexia in children.

How to take them

☑ **DOSAGE:** *For heart disease, Raynaud's disease, lupus and psoriasis:* Take 3000 mg of fish oils a day. *For rheumatoid arthritis:* Take 6000 mg a day. *For inflammatory bowel disease:* Take 5000 mg a day.

◐ **GUIDELINES FOR USE:** Fish oil supplements are not necessary for heart disease prevention or treatment if you eat oily fish at least twice a week. However, supplements are recommended for rheumatoid arthritis and other inflammatory conditions. Take capsules with meals. Supplements may be easier to tolerate if you take them in divided doses: for example, 1000 mg three times a day, instead of 3000 mg at one time. When taking supplementary fish oil, ensure that you get extra antioxidant protection by eating plenty of fruit and vegetables or taking extra vitamin E.

Possible side effects

Fish oil capsules may cause belching, flatulence, bloating, nausea and diarrhoea. Very high doses may result in a slightly fishy body odour. There is some concern that high doses can lead to internal bleeding, but a study of people with heart disease who took 8000 mg of fish oil supplements in addition to aspirin (an anticoagulant) found no increase in the incidence of internal bleeding. Some studies have found that high doses of fish oils worsen blood sugar control in people with diabetes; others have shown no effect. To be safe, diabetics should not take more than 2000 mg of fish oil supplements a day except on medical advice.

Individuals with high levels of triglycerides should be careful if they also have high LDL ('bad') cholesterol: therapeutic doses of fish oils can increase LDL. Garlic supplements may be the remedy. One study found that garlic reversed the fish oils' LDL-raising effect. For rheumatoid arthritis and other inflammatory conditions, eating fish is probably not sufficient, and fish-oil supplements are recommended.

RECENT FINDINGS

A study involving 120 children in County Durham found that supplements of omega-3s can help to improve the reading and writing abilities and concentration of children with learning difficulties.

～～

Fish oils may help to prevent breast cancer. A French study indicated that women with a high intake of omega-3s had a significantly reduced risk of breast cancer. Further work suggested that omega-3s may increase the production of one of the genes that is known to suppress breast cancer.

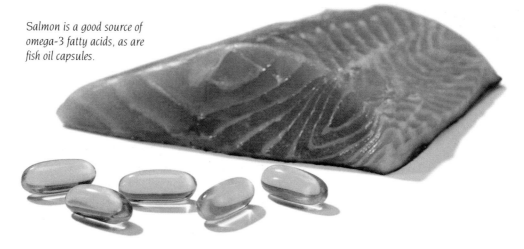

Salmon is a good source of omega-3 fatty acids, as are fish oil capsules.

5-HTP

People suffering from depression, insomnia, migraines or obesity have a new supplement to consider: 5-HTP. Unlike the amino acid tryptophan, which was recalled owing to safety concerns, 5-HTP appears to be safe – and it may be even more effective than its close chemical cousin.

Common uses

- *Relieves depression.*
- *Helps to overcome insomnia.*
- *Aids in weight control.*
- *Treats migraines.*
- *May ease pain of fibromyalgia.*

Forms

- Capsule
- Tablet

What it is

The nutrient 5-HTP, short for 5-hydroxytryptophan, is a derivative of the amino acid tryptophan which is found in such high-protein foods as beef, chicken, fish and dairy products. The body makes 5-HTP from the tryptophan present in our diets. Tryptophan is also found in the seeds of an African plant called *Griffonia simplicifolia*, which is the source of the 5-HTP supplements sold in health-food shops.

The focus of much recent interest, 5-HTP acts on the brain, helping to elevate mood, promote sleep, aid weight loss and relieve migraines, among other uses. Unlike many other supplements (and drugs) that contain substances with molecules too large to pass from the bloodstream into the brain, 5-HTP is small enough to enter the brain. Once there it is converted into a vital nervous-system chemical, or neurotransmitter, called serotonin. Although it affects many parts of the body, serotonin's most important actions take place in the brain, where it influences everything from mood to appetite to sleep.

Its close relationship with the amino acid tryptophan makes 5-HTP somewhat controversial. In 1989 the sale of L-tryptophan and other tryptophan supplements was banned in the UK and other countries after reports of a fatal illness among those taking it. The illness was later found to be caused by contamination of the supplement during the manufacturing process, not by the tryptophan itself. In 1994 5-HTP began to be sold in the USA as an over-the-counter alternative to tryptophan, and it is now available in the UK. 5-HTP is not made in the same way as tryptophan, and so it avoids the contamination problems of its predecessor. Though safety concerns have been raised, many researchers believe it is safe and effective.

What it does

In recent years 5-HTP has been studied as a treatment for such mood disorders as depression, anxiety and panic attacks because it can boost levels of serotonin in the brain. Scientists are also investigating whether

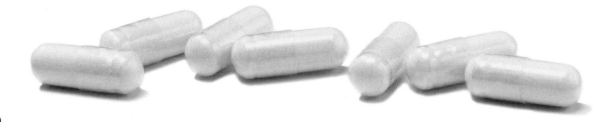

it may work for an array of additional complaints linked to low serotonin levels, including migraines, fibromyalgia, obesity, eating disorders, PMS and even violent behaviour. Although additional research is needed to determine its effectiveness against many of these conditions, preliminary studies suggest it may be very beneficial for some.

✦ **MAJOR BENEFITS:** For decades doctors have been prescribing 5-HTP for the treatment of depression and insomnia. In some cases it may be more effective, lift depression more quickly and produce fewer side effects than standard antidepressant drugs. In one study, more than half the patients with long-term depression who were resistant to all other antidepressants felt better after taking 5-HTP. The nutrient has also been shown to promote sleep, and to improve the quality of sleep, by increasing the amount of time people spend in two key sleep stages: deep sleep and REM sleep (the dreaming stage). After dreaming for longer, those on 5-HTP awaken feeling more rested and refreshed.

✦ **ADDITIONAL BENEFITS:** Individuals trying to lose weight or suffering from migraines may benefit from 5-HTP. In one study, overweight women who took the supplement ate fewer calories, lost more weight and were more likely to feel full while on a diet than those given a placebo. It may also be useful in relieving severe headaches, including migraines, reducing not only their frequency but also their intensity and duration.

The supplement may also work to increase pain tolerance in those with fibromyalgia, a chronic condition marked by aches and fatigue, in part by helping to relieve any underlying depression. In an Italian study of 200 fibromyalgia sufferers, those who took 5-HTP with conventional antidepressants had less pain than those taking either 5-HTP or the drugs alone. If you are taking antidepressants, don't try 5-HTP without consulting your doctor first: adverse reactions can occur.

How to take it

⊘ **DOSAGE:** The recommended dose for depression and most other ailments is 50 to 100 mg three times a day. *For migraines:* Take up to 100 mg three times a day if necessary. *For insomnia:* Take a single 100 mg dose half an hour before bedtime. When using 5-HTP it is advisable to start with a low dose (such as 50 mg) and gradually increase it if needed.

◉ **GUIDELINES FOR USE:** To ensure rapid absorption, take 5-HTP on an empty stomach. For weight control, take the supplement 30 minutes before meals. Don't use 5-HTP for more than three months except on medical advice. Some doctors combine it with the mood-enhancing herb St John's wort, but you should not take it with that herb or with conventional antidepressants without checking with your doctor first.

Possible side effects

The generally mild side effects include nausea, constipation, flatulence, drowsiness and a reduced sex drive. Nausea usually diminishes within a few days.

Flaxseed oil

A rich source of healing oil, flaxseed (or linseed) has been cultivated for more than 7000 years. The oil is used to prevent and treat heart disease and to relieve a variety of inflammatory disorders and hormone-related problems, including infertility.

Linum usitatissimum

Common uses

- Helps to protect against heart disease.
- Promotes healthy skin, hair and nails.
- May reduce inflammation.
- May be useful for infertility, impotence, menstrual cramps and endometriosis.
- May help to alleviate nerve disorders.
- Relieves constipation and diverticular disorders.

Forms

- Capsule
- Oil
- Powder
- Softgel

What it is

The flax plant was first used as a fibre for weaving – and it remains the source of natural linen fabric. However, it has also been renowned for centuries for its medicinal properties. The slender annual grows up to a metre in height and bears blue flowers from February to September. Both the oil from the seeds (also known as linseeds) and the seeds themselves are used for therapeutic purposes.

What it does

Flaxseeds are a source of essential fatty acids (EFAs) – fats and oils critical for health which the body cannot make on its own. One EFA found in flaxseeds, alpha-linolenic acid, is known as an omega-3 fatty acid; it is also found in many other seed oils, including rape, soya, blackcurrant and walnut. However, alpha-linolenic acid is not as potent as the omega-3 fatty acids found in fish oils, which have been acclaimed in recent years for protecting against heart disease and for treating many other ailments.

Flaxseeds also contain omega-6 fatty acids (in the form of linolenic acid), the same healthy fats that are present in many vegetable oils. In addition, flaxseeds provide substances called lignans which appear to have beneficial effects on various hormones and may help to fight cancer, bacteria, viruses and fungi. Weight for weight, flaxseeds contain up to 800 times the lignans found in most other foods.

✪ **MAJOR BENEFITS:** EFAs work throughout the body to protect cell membranes – the outer coverings that are gatekeepers for all cells,

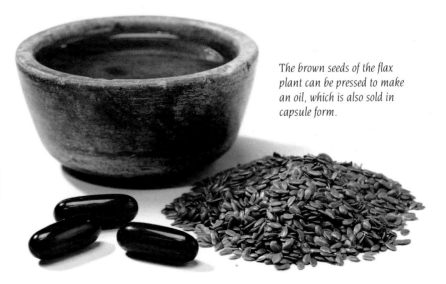

The brown seeds of the flax plant can be pressed to make an oil, which is also sold in capsule form.

admitting healthy nutrients and barring damaging substances. That function explains why flaxseed oil may have such far-reaching effects.

Flaxseed oil works to lower cholesterol, and so protects against heart disease. It may also prove beneficial against angina and high blood pressure. A recent five-year study at Simmons College in Boston, Massachusetts, indicated that it might be useful in preventing second heart attacks. As a digestive aid it can prevent or even dissolve gallstones, and it also promotes healthy hair and nails. In addition it may facilitate the transmission of nerve impulses, which makes it potentially useful for numbness and tingling as well as for chronic brain and nerve ailments such as Alzheimer's disease, or nerve damage from diabetes. It may help to fight fatigue, but more research is needed.

Crushed flaxseeds are an excellent natural source of fibre. They add bulk to stools, and their oil lubricates the stools, making flaxseeds useful for the relief of constipation and diverticular complaints.

✦ **ADDITIONAL BENEFITS:** Flaxseeds contain plant-based oestrogens, called phytoestrogens, which mimic the female sex hormone oestrogen, so the oil can have beneficial effects on the menstrual cycle, balancing the ratio of oestrogen to progesterone. It helps to improve uterine function and can therefore treat fertility problems. It may help to reduce menopausal symptoms such as hot flushes. Also, possibly because of anti-inflammatory action, flaxseed oil can reduce menstrual cramps or the pain of fibrocystic breasts.

The oil can promote well-being in men as well: it has shown some promise in treating male infertility and prostate problems. In some studies flaxseeds were also found to possess antibacterial, antifungal and antiviral properties, which may partly explain why flaxseed oil is effective against ailments such as cold sores and shingles.

How to take it

◨ **DOSAGE:** Liquid flaxseed oil is the easiest way to take a therapeutic amount, which ranges from 1 teaspoon to 1 tablespoon once or twice a day. For the equivalent of 1 tablespoon of the oil in capsule form you need to swallow about 14 capsules, each containing 1000 mg of oil. For flaxseed fibre, mix 1 or 2 tablespoons of ground flaxseeds with a glass of water and drink it up to three times a day; the treatment may take a day or so to be effective.

◨ **GUIDELINES FOR USE:** Take flaxseed oil with food, which enhances absorption by the body. You can also mix it with juice, yoghurt, cottage cheese or other foods and drinks.

Possible side effects

Flaxseed oil appears to be very safe. Those using the ground seeds may experience some flatulence initially, but this should soon disappear.

Folic acid

Folic acid is necessary for every function in the body that requires cell multiplication. It is especially important in foetal development, and helps to produce key chemicals for the brain and nervous system. Yet nine out of ten adults consume too little of this vital nutrient.

Common uses

- Protects against birth defects.
- Reduces heart disease and stroke risk.
- Lowers risk for several cancers.
- Can alleviate depression, especially in elderly people.

Forms

- Capsule
- Liquid
- Powder
- Tablet

CAUTION!

Folic acid supplements may mask a type of anaemia caused by a vitamin B_{12} deficiency. Unchecked, this anaemia can cause irreversible nerve damage and dementia. If you take folic acid supplements, be sure to take extra vitamin B_{12} as well.

REMINDER: If you have a medical or psychiatric condition, consult your doctor before taking supplements.

What it is

A water-soluble B vitamin, also called folacin or folate, folic acid was identified in the 1940s, when it was extracted from spinach. The body cannot store it for very long, so you need to replenish your supply daily. Cooking, or even long storage, can destroy up to half the folic acid in foods, so supplements may be the best way to ensure that your body is getting enough.

What it does

Folic acid is utilised in the body thousands of times a day to make blood cells, heal wounds, build muscle – and in every other process that requires cell division. Folic acid is critical to DNA and RNA formation and ensures that cells duplicate normally.

PREVENTION: Adequate folic acid at conception and for the first three months of pregnancy greatly reduces the risk of serious birth defects, including spina bifida and cleft palate, so women should take folic acid if they are trying to conceive as well as during pregnancy. The B vitamin appears to regulate the body's production and use of homocysteine, an amino acid-like substance that at high levels may damage the lining of blood vessels, making them more susceptible to plaque build-up. This makes folic acid an important weapon against heart disease. It may also ward off cancers, especially those of the lungs, cervix, colon and rectum.

ADDITIONAL BENEFITS: People who are depressed often suffer from a deficiency of folic acid. Supplements of the B vitamin may relieve depression by reducing homocysteine, high levels of which are believed to contribute to the condition. Studies also show that taking folic acid improves the effectiveness of antidepressants in people with low folic

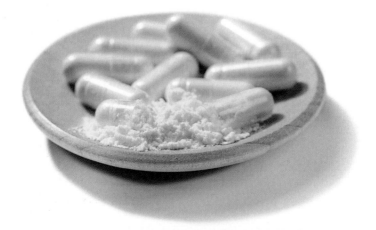

acid levels. Folic acid supplements have been useful in treating gout and irritable bowel syndrome as well. High homocysteine levels are thought to be a factor in the development of osteoporosis, so folic acid may even help to keep bones strong.

How much you need

The current recommended target for folic acid is 200 mcg a day for adults, but women who are pregnant or likely to become pregnant are advised to take 400 mcg daily, in addition to the recommended dietary target of 200 mcg daily. Supplements are important for older people, who may not get enough of the vitamin in food.

⊟ **IF YOU GET TOO LITTLE:** Though relatively rare, a severe folic acid deficiency can cause a form of anaemia (megaloblastic anaemia), a sore red tongue, chronic diarrhoea and poor growth (in children). Alcoholics and people who are on certain medications (for cancer or epilepsy) or who have malabsorption diseases (Crohn's, coeliac, sprue) are susceptible to severe deficiency. Much more common is a low level of folic acid, which causes no symptoms but raises the risk of heart disease or birth defects.

⊕ **IF YOU GET TOO MUCH:** Very large doses – 5000 to 10,000 mcg – offer no benefit and may be dangerous for people with hormone-related cancers, such as those of the breast or prostate. High doses may also cause seizures in those with epilepsy. The advised upper safe limit for folic acid in the UK is 1000 mcg for adults.

How to take it

☑ **DOSAGE:** *For overall good health and the prevention of heart disease:* Take a dose of 200 mcg of folic acid a day. *For pregnant women and women who might become pregnant:* Take 400 mcg a day. (Adequate folic acid stores are important because the vitamin plays a role in a baby's development from conception.) *For people with depression:* Take 400 mcg a day, as part of a vitamin B-complex supplement.

◉ **GUIDELINES FOR USE:** Folic acid can be taken at any time of the day, with or without food. When taking individual folic acid supplements for any reason, combine it with an additional 1000 mcg of vitamin B_{12} to prevent a B_{12} deficiency.

Other sources

Excellent food sources of folic acid include green vegetables, beans, whole grains and orange juice. Some refined grain products are now fortified with folic acid.

RECENT FINDINGS

For prevention of disease, the best way to obtain enough folic acid may be through supplements. In a small study, people taking 400 mcg of folic acid a day in pills or in specially fortified foods increased their folic acid level. But those who just ate foods naturally rich in folic acid showed no increase. Scientists speculate that the folic acid found naturally in foods may not be absorbed well enough to have a therapeutic effect.

A preliminary study by Oxford University hints that folic acid may play a role in preventing Alzheimer's disease. People with the disease tended to have lower blood levels of folic acid and vitamin B_{12} than healthy people of the same age.

DID YOU KNOW?

To get the daily 200 mcg of folic acid recommended for good health, you'd need to eat 12 spears of asparagus a day.

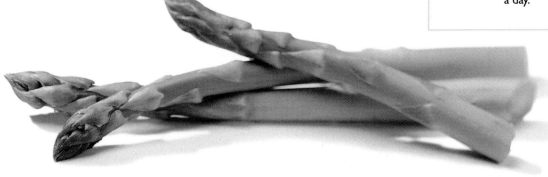

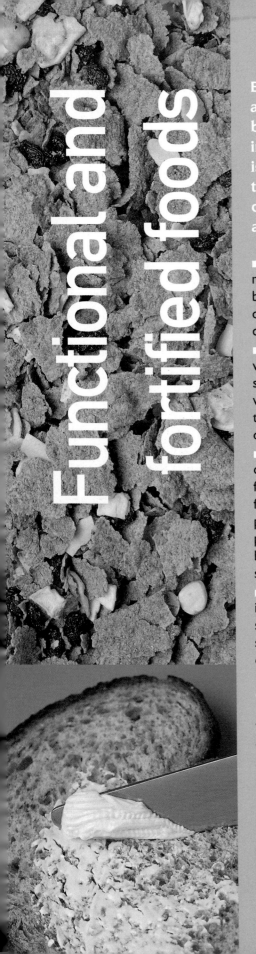

Enhanced foods – such as bioyoghurts and cereals with added nutrients – are growing in popularity. Some can boost vitamin and mineral levels; others show promise in preventing or treating ailments, but more research is needed to prove their worth. The big advantage of these 'functional' or 'fortified' foods lies in the amounts of 'macronutrients', such as calcium and omega-3 fatty acids, that they contain – much more than tablets.

■ Functional foods are foods meant to offer a specific health benefit over and above the level of nutrients found in their conventional counterparts.

■ Fortified foods have had extra vitamins and/or minerals added so that one portion of the food will provide a high percentage of the recommended daily intake of that nutrient.

■ Many fortified foods can be considered functional foods – for example, bread fortified with folic acid, which may help to prevent heart disease and protect women from having babies with neural-tube defects such as spina bifida.

■ Examples of functional foods include bioyoghurts containing specially selected bacteria, and spreads with added fish oils or cholesterol-lowering agents.

CAN FOODS ACT AS MEDICINES?

The purpose of 'enhancing' foods is to aid in the prevention of certain diseases, or in the treatment of certain conditions. For example, 'friendly' bacteria are used to help to relieve bowel problems, and plant sterols to reduce cholesterol levels. However, functional foods are categorised as foods rather than medicines, so under food labelling law no claims that they 'prevent' or 'cure' specific diseases can be made for them.

REGULAR INTAKE

To be effective, functional foods must be taken regularly, just like dietary supplements. Some manufacturers are producing functional foods with the same nutritional objective but in different formats, in order to provide variety in the diet.

PROBIOTICS AND PREBIOTICS

The gut contains billions of bacteria. These play a vital role in the normal functioning of the digestive system, the lowering of blood cholesterol levels, the promotion of the immune response, protection from colon cancer, and the synthesis of certain vitamins. They also prevent colonisation of the gut by harmful bacteria that may cause food poisoning.

Stress, antibiotics, certain drugs and female hormones can cause a proliferation of disease-causing bacteria at the expense of numbers of the bacteria that keep us healthy. However, the balance of microbes in the intestines may be improved by taking probiotics: probably the most widely available functional foods.

Probiotics come in the form of bioyoghurts, milk-based drinks – such as Yakult and Actimel – and fruit juices with added 'friendly' bacteria. The most commonly used friendly bacteria are the lactobacilli (acidophilus) and bifido-bacteria (bifidus) families. To be effective they may have to be eaten daily, or the improved colonisation of the gut may not be sustained.

Prebiotics – also used to improve intestinal health – are carbohydrates that pass unchanged through the digestive system and enter the large bowel, where they act as nutrients for 'friendly' bacteria, including those that may have been taken in probiotics.

The 'friendly' bacteria are then able to compete more success-fully against the harmful micro-organisms, resulting in a healthier gut function.

PHYTOESTROGENS

High intakes of isoflavones, the most active phytoestrogens in the human diet (see *page 135*), may reduce the risk of coronary heart disease and some cancers, including breast, prostate and bowel cancer. They may also help to reduce menopausal symptoms and the risk of osteoporosis. Functional foods containing soya protein or the pure isoflavones are being developed.

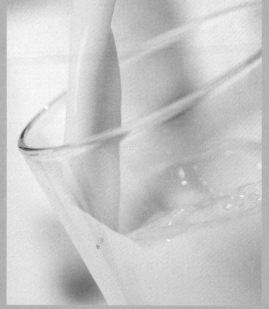

PLANT STEROLS

A group of plant chemicals with a structure similar to cholesterol is plant sterols. They are not absorbed by the gut, but have been found to reduce the absorption of cholesterol both from foods and from the bile that the liver dis-charges into the intestine.

Plant sterols can lower blood cholesterol levels and thereby reduce the risk of heart disease. For this reason they are added to some margarines and sold as functional foods; a certain amount of the margarine must be eaten each day for the desired effect to be achieved.

FOLIC ACID

A low folic acid intake has been linked to increased blood levels of homocysteine, and possibly to incidence of cancer of the colon and Alzheimer's disease.

Homocysteine is a product of protein metabolism found in the blood; in some people its level can rise, and this is believed to increase the risk of heart disease. Levels of homocysteine are usually controlled by three enzymes, two of which are dependent on the presence of folic acid, or folate.

Many foods, such as bread and breakfast cereals, are fortified with this B vitamin to help to reduce the incidence of these diseases and to protect unborn babies from developing neural-tube defects.

FISH OILS

Fish oils containing omega-3 essential fatty acids (EFAs) have been shown to reduce both the risk of death following a heart attack and the incidence of heart disease. Intakes of omega-3 EFAs in the European Union are currently at only 50% of recommended levels.

Margarines enriched with fish oils have been available in the UK, but did not prove popular. Manufacturers are developing other foods rich in omega-3 fats, but masking their taste is a major problem.

BONE HEALTH

Calcium, magnesium and vitamin D are believed to be the most important nutrients for bone health. For decades white flour has been fortified with calcium, and margarines fortified with vitamin D. Functional foods containing nutrients to aid bone health have also now become available. They include fortified orange juice, cereal bars and chocolate drinks.

Fungi

Ganoderma lucidum (reishi)
Grifola frondosa (maitake)
Lentinus edodes (shiitake)

Common uses

- *Build immunity.*
- *Help to prevent cancer.*
- *Enhance cancer treatments.*
- *Alleviate bronchitis, sinusitis.*
- *Treat chronic fatigue syndrome.*
- *Help to prevent heart disease.*

Forms

- Capsule
- Dried mushrooms
- Fresh mushrooms
- Liquid
- Powder
- Tablet
- Tea

CAUTION!

■ If you are taking anticoagulant drugs, it is advisable to avoid reishi supplements because the mushrooms contain compounds that also 'thin' the blood.

REMINDER: If you have a medical condition, consult your doctor before taking supplements.

Shiitake and maitake are more than just exotic-sounding items on a Japanese menu. In fact, they are members of a special group of medicinal fungi, or mushrooms, that have been heralded in Asia for centuries as longevity tonics and immune-system boosters.

What they are

Traditional Asian medicine has long cherished certain species of mushroom – including maitake, reishi and shiitake – for their health-promoting effects. Reishi mushrooms, in particular, are one of the major Chinese tonics, and were first described in Chinese writings of 200 BC. Although other mushrooms – tree ear and oyster mushrooms, for instance – may also provide some health benefits, most research has focused on the three types mentioned above.

The mushrooms are available as powders (in loose form, to be brewed as a tea, or in capsules or tablets) or as liquid extracts, in which their potency is concentrated. Dried reishi and fresh and dried shiitake and maitake mushrooms may be found in Asian supermarkets and in some gourmet shops, but for therapeutic purposes supplements are preferred. Maitake, reishi and shiitake mushroom powders are sometimes combined in one capsule.

What they do

Medicinal mushrooms have various effects, including boosting the body's immune system, lowering cholesterol, acting as an anticoagulant and playing a supportive role in the treatment of cancer.

⊛ **MAJOR BENEFITS:** Maitake mushrooms are commonly used in Japan to strengthen the immune systems of people undergoing chemotherapy treatment for cancer. Studies have shown that maitake extracts increase the effectiveness of lower chemotherapy doses while protecting healthy cells from the damage such drugs can cause.

Medicinal mushrooms boost the immune system, aiding in the battle against disease-causing organisms. Some studies show that they may be powerful enough to help people with HIV infection and AIDS, who have very weak immune systems. For example, shiitake mushrooms contain a carbohydrate compound called lentinan, which promotes the body's production of T cells and other immune-system components. Other people with compromised immune systems, such as those with chronic fatigue syndrome, may benefit from medicinal mushrooms too.

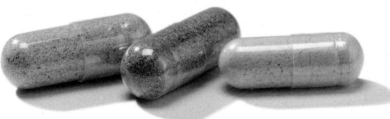

Supplements made from shiitake, reishi and maitake mushrooms (left to right) come in capsule form.

ADDITIONAL BENEFITS: Traditionally, reishi mushrooms (known to the Chinese as 'spirit plants') are used to encourage relaxation, which makes them suitable for the treatment of stress and fatigue. Reishi also contain anti-inflammatory compounds that are beneficial for bronchitis and possibly for other respiratory ailments. In a Chinese study of 2000 people with bronchitis, 60% to 90% of those given reishi tablets improved within two weeks. Maitake, reishi and shiitake mushrooms may also help to fight heart disease by reducing the tendency of blood to clot, lowering blood pressure and possibly reducing cholesterol levels.

How to take them

DOSAGE: *For immune-system support for cancer:* Take 200 mg maitake, 500 mg of reishi and 400 mg shiitake mushrooms three times a day. For *heart disease or* HIV/AIDS: Take 1500 mg of reishi and 600 mg maitake daily. For *bronchitis or sinusitis:* Take 1500 mg of reishi and/or 600 mg of maitake daily during the illness.

GUIDELINES FOR USE: The effects of medicinal mushrooms are not dramatic, and may need several months to become apparent. For best results, divide the supplements into two or three daily doses and take with or without food. As these medicinal mushrooms are also traditional foods, the dried fungi can be added to soups or infused with hot water to make teas. Reishi mushrooms occur in six different colours; the red and purple varieties are most commonly used medicinally.

Possible side effects

Maitake, reishi and shiitake mushrooms are all safe when used in appropriate doses. In rare cases, long-term use of reishi – three to six months of daily use – may cause dryness in the mouth, a skin rash and itchiness, an upset stomach, nosebleeds or bloody stools. If any of these symptoms occur, stop taking reishi. Pregnant or breastfeeding women should consult a doctor before trying any of the mushrooms medicinally.

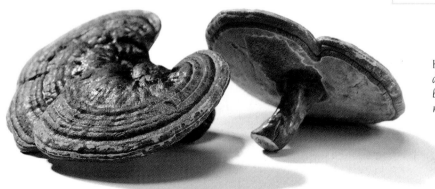

Helpful in combating stress, dried reishi mushrooms can be simmered in water to make a calming tea.

Garlic

Allium sativum

Prized by the ancient Egyptians for its strength-enhancing properties, garlic has since been used to treat every type of ailment, from leprosy to haemorrhoids. Modern research has focused on exploiting its potential to reduce the risk of heart disease and cancer.

Common uses

- May lower cholesterol levels.
- Reduces blood clotting.
- Fights infections.
- Acts to boost immunity.
- May prevent some cancers.
- May produce a slight drop in blood pressure.
- Combats fungal infections.

Forms

- Capsule
- Fresh herb
- Liquid
- Oil
- Powder
- Softgel
- Tablet

CAUTION!

- Consult your doctor if you are taking drugs to prevent blood clots (anticoagulants or aspirin) or to reduce high blood pressure (antihypertensives). Garlic may intensify the effects of these drugs.

REMINDER: *If you have a medical condition, consult your doctor before taking supplements.*

What it is

For thousands of years garlic has been valued for its therapeutic powers. Egyptian pyramid builders took it for strength and endurance; in the 19th century Louis Pasteur investigated its antibacterial properties; and physicians in the two world wars used it to treat battle wounds. Garlic is related to the onion, the shallot and other plants in the genus *Allium*. The entire plant is odoriferous, but the strongest aroma is concentrated in the bulb, the site of garlic's healing powers and flavour.

Most of garlic's health benefits derive from its more than 100 sulphur compounds. When the bulb is crushed or chewed, alliin, one of these compounds, becomes allicin, the chemical responsible for garlic's odour and health-giving effects. In turn, some of the allicin is rapidly broken down into other sulphur compounds, such as ajoene, which can also have medicinal properties. Cooking garlic inhibits the formation of allicin and eliminates some of the other therapeutic chemicals.

What it does

Traditionally, garlic has been employed to treat a wide range of ailments and diseases. Today researchers are focusing on its potential to reduce the risk of heart disease and cancer.

PREVENTION: The liberal use of garlic in Mediterranean cooking may partly explain why countries such as Italy and Spain have such a low incidence of hardening of the arteries (atherosclerosis).

Several studies suggest that garlic can prevent heart disease in various ways. For example, garlic makes platelets (the cells involved in blood clotting) less likely to clump and stick to artery walls, and so reduces the risk of a heart attack. There is evidence that the herb dissolves clot-forming proteins which can affect plaque development. Garlic also lowers blood pressure slightly, mainly through its ability to widen blood vessels and help blood to circulate more freely. Results of recent studies examining garlic's effect on cholesterol are not clear-cut,

Garlic supplements come in many forms, including capsules, tablets and softgels.

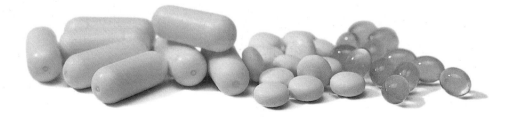

but most doctors who favour nutritional remedies think that garlic, perhaps in combination with other cholesterol-lowering supplements, is worth a try. The herb may affect the metabolism of cholesterol in the liver; as a result, less cholesterol is released into the blood.

ADDITIONAL BENEFITS: Garlic may have anticancer properties. It has been found to be particularly effective in preventing digestive cancers and possibly even breast and prostate cancers, but is not clear how garlic produces these benefits. Several mechanisms may be involved; for example, the herb acts to increase the level of enzymes that can detoxify cancer triggers. Garlic also blocks the formation of nitrites linked to stomach cancer, and it stimulates the immune system. Its antioxidant properties are important as well.

Garlic is often effective against infectious organisms – viruses, bacteria and fungi – because allicin can block the enzymes that give the organisms their ability to invade and damage tissues. The herb has also been shown to inhibit the fungi responsible for athlete's foot and swimmer's ear.

How to take it

DOSAGE: Look for supplements that supply 4000 mcg of allicin potential per tablet, approximately the same amount of allicin potential found in one clove of fresh garlic. *For general health or to help high cholesterol*: Take a 400 to 600 mg garlic supplement each day. *For colds and flu*: Take a 400 to 600 mg garlic supplement four times a day. *For topical benefits*: Apply garlic oil two or three times a day. Some skin conditions, including warts and insect bites, may respond to garlic oil, or a crushed raw garlic clove, applied directly to the affected area.

GUIDELINES FOR USE: Garlic can be taken indefinitely. However, if you are using the herb for cholesterol problems, have your levels checked after three months to see if they have changed; if you have derived no benefits from garlic, talk to your doctor about other remedies.

Possible side effects

Some people develop indigestion, intestinal gas and diarrhoea when taking high doses of garlic. Using enteric-coated supplements may reduce such side effects. Skin rashes have also been reported.

To get the full medicinal benefits of fresh garlic, it should be eaten raw.

Ginger

Zingiber officinale

From ancient India and China to Greece and Rome, ginger was revered as a culinary and medicinal spice. Medieval Europeans traced the herb to the Garden of Eden. Valued by traditional healers, ginger is still widely used to prevent motion sickness and as a remedy for digestive problems.

Common uses

- *Alleviates nausea and dizziness.*
- *May relieve the pain and inflammation of arthritis.*
- *Eases muscle aches.*
- *Relieves cold and flu symptoms.*
- *Reduces flatulence.*

Forms

- Capsule
- Crystallised herb
- Fresh or dried root/tea
- Liquid
- Oil
- Softgel
- Tablet
- Tincture

CAUTION!

■ Up to 250 mg of ginger four times a day may relieve morning sickness during the first two months of pregnancy, but higher doses or longer use require medical supervision.

■ Chemotherapy patients should not take ginger on an empty stomach because it can irritate the stomach lining.

REMINDER: If you have a medical condition, consult your doctor before taking supplements.

What it is

Renowned for its stomach-settling properties, ginger is native to parts of India and China as well as Jamaica and other tropical areas. This warm-climate perennial is closely related to turmeric and cardamom, and its roots are used for culinary and therapeutic purposes. As a spice, ginger adds a hot and lemony flavour to foods as disparate as biscuits and roast pork. Medicinally, it continues to play a major role in traditional healing.

What it does

For thousands of years, all around the globe, this pungent spice has been popular as a treatment for digestive problems ranging from mild indigestion and flatulence to nausea and vomiting. It has also been used to relieve colds and arthritis. Modern research into ginger's active ingredients confirms the effectiveness of many of these ancient remedies.

MAJOR BENEFITS: What can you do with a seasick sailor? The answer is: try ginger. In a Danish study a group of 40 naval cadets took 1 gram of powdered ginger a day; they were much less likely to break out in a cold sweat and to vomit (classic symptoms of seasickness) than were 39 others who took a placebo.

Ginger works primarily in the digestive tract, boosting digestive fluids and neutralising acids, so it is sometimes used as an alternative to antinausea drugs that can affect the central nervous system and cause grogginess. Studies of women undergoing exploratory surgery (laparoscopy) or major gynaecological surgery show that taking 1 gram of ginger before an operation can significantly reduce postoperative nausea and vomiting, a common side effect of anaesthetics and other drugs used in surgery. Ginger also appears to counter the nausea created by chemotherapy, though it is advisable to take it with food to minimise any stomach irritation.

Ginger's antinausea effects make it useful for reducing dizziness, a common problem in older patients, as well as for treating morning sickness. For years ginger has been a staple of folk medicine, primarily as a digestive aid to counter stomach upset. Ginger supplements (or fresh pulp mixed with lime juice) are also a good remedy for flatulence.

ADDITIONAL BENEFITS: Ginger's anti-inflammatory and pain-relieving properties may help to relieve the muscle aches and chronic pain associated with arthritis. In a study of seven women with rheumatoid arthritis (an autoimmune disease characterised by severe inflammation) a daily dose of just 5 to 50 grams of fresh ginger or capsules containing up to 1 gram of powdered ginger was shown to lessen joint pain and inflammation. Its anti-inflammatory properties suggest that ginger may ease bronchial constriction brought on by colds or flu.

How to take it

☑ **Dosage:** *To prevent motion sickness, dizziness and nausea, reduce flatulence, and relieve chronic pain or rheumatoid arthritis*: Take ginger up to three times a day, or every four hours as needed. The usual dose is 100 to 200 mg of standardised extract in capsule or tablet form, or 1 or 2 grams of fresh powdered ginger, or a 1.25 cm slice of fresh ginger root. Other preparations, including ginger tea, can be used several times a day for similar purposes and for arthritis and pain relief. Ginger tea is available in tea bags, or you can add ½ teaspoon of grated ginger root to a cup of very hot water. On journeys, try crystallised ginger: a 2.5 cm square, about ½ cm thick, contains approximately 500 mg of ginger. *For aching muscles*: Rub several drops of ginger oil, mixed with a tablespoon of almond oil or another neutral oil, on the sore areas. *For relief of colds and flu*: Drink up to four cups of ginger tea a day as needed to reduce symptoms.

◉ **Guidelines for use:** Taking large doses on an empty stomach may lead to indigestion: take with food, and take ginger capsules with fluid. To prevent motion sickness, ginger should be taken three to four hours before your departure, and then every four hours as needed, up to four times a day. For postoperative nausea, begin taking ginger the day before your operation, under medical supervision.

Possible side effects

Ginger is very safe for a broad range of complaints, whether it is taken in a concentrated capsule form, eaten fresh or sipped as a tea or ginger ale. Occasional indigestion seems to be the only documented side effect.

Whether eaten fresh or taken in the form of capsules, ginger is a potent remedy for nausea and dizziness.

DID YOU KNOW?

A cup of ginger tea contains the equivalent of about 250 mg of the powdered herb. A heavily spiced Chinese or Indian ginger dish has about twice that amount.

FACTS & TIPS

■ The ancient Greeks prized ginger so highly as an aid to digestion that they mixed it into their bread, creating the first gingerbread.

■ To ease the aches and chest tightness associated with colds and flu, many folk-healers recommend chewing fresh ginger, drinking ginger tea, or squeezing juice from ginger root into a spoonful of honey.

Ginkgo biloba

Ginkgo biloba

This popular herbal medicine, derived from one of the oldest species of tree on earth, is widely marketed as a memory booster. Ginkgo biloba does help to combat age-related memory loss, but whether it is a 'smart pill' meant for everyone remains to be seen.

Common uses

- *May slow down the progression of Alzheimer's symptoms; sharpens concentration and memory, particularly in elderly people.*
- *Lessens depression and anxiety in some elderly people.*
- *Alleviates coldness in the extremities (Raynaud's disease) and painful leg cramps (intermittent claudication).*
- *Relieves headaches, tinnitus (ringing in the ears) and dizziness.*
- *May restore erections in men with impotence.*

Forms

- Capsule
- Liquid
- Powder
- Softgel
- Tablet
- Tincture

What it is

The medicinal form of the herb is extracted from the fan-shaped leaves of the ancient ginkgo biloba tree, a species that has survived in China for more than 200 million years. A concentrated form of the herb, known as ginkgo biloba extract, or GBE, is used to make the supplement. Commonly called ginkgo, GBE is obtained by drying and milling the leaves and then extracting the active ingredients in a mixture of acetone and water.

What it does

Ginkgo may have beneficial effects on both the circulatory and the central nervous systems. It increases blood flow to the arms and legs and the brain by regulating the tone and elasticity of blood vessels, from the largest arteries to the tiniest capillaries. It also acts like aspirin by helping to reduce the 'stickiness' of the blood, thereby lowering the risk of blood clots. Ginkgo appears to have antioxidant properties as well, mopping up the damaging compounds known as free radicals and aiding in the maintenance of healthy blood cells. Some researchers report that it enhances the nervous system by promoting the delivery of additional oxygen and blood sugar (glucose) to nerve cells.

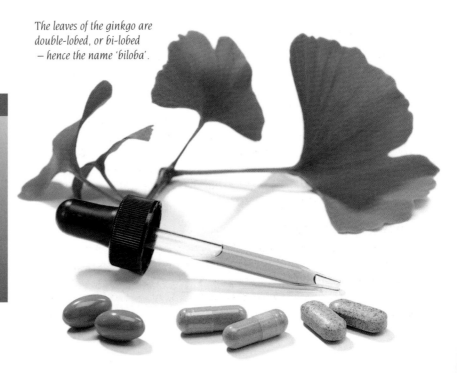

The leaves of the ginkgo are double-lobed, or bi-lobed – hence the name 'biloba'.

PREVENTION: Modern interest in ginkgo centres on the herb's potential as a preventative for age-related memory loss. There is also an indication that ginkgo may make healthy people better able to focus their thoughts or to remember. So far it is those people who are already suffering from diminished blood flow to the brain who have benefited most from taking the herb. Current research is trying to determine whether ginkgo's ability to prevent blood clots may stave off heart attacks or strokes.

MAJOR BENEFITS: The fact that ginkgo aids blood flow to the brain – thereby increasing its oxygen supply – is particularly important to elderly people whose arteries may have narrowed with cholesterol build-up or other conditions. Diminished blood flow has been linked to Alzheimer's disease and memory loss, as well as to anxiety, headaches, depression, confusion, tinnitus and dizziness. All may be helped by ginkgo.

ADDITIONAL BENEFITS: Ginkgo also promotes blood flow to the arms and legs, which makes it useful for reducing the pain, cramping and weakness caused by narrowed arteries in the leg, a disorder called intermittent claudication. There are indications that the herb may improve circulation to the extremities in people with Raynaud's disease, and help victims of scleroderma, a rare autoimmune disorder.

In addition some research suggests that, by increasing blood flow to the nerve fibres of the eyes and ears, ginkgo may be of value in treating macular degeneration or diabetes-related eye disease (both leading causes of blindness) as well as some types of hearing loss.

Other studies are in progress to assess the possible effectiveness of ginkgo in speeding up recovery from certain strokes and head injuries, as well as in treating other conditions that may be related to circulatory or nervous system impairment, including impotence, multiple sclerosis and nerve damage linked to diabetes. Before the introduction of leaf extracts, traditional Chinese healers used ginkgo nuts for treating asthma because they appear to alleviate wheezing and other respiratory complaints.

How to take it

DOSAGE: Use supplements that contain ginkgo biloba extract, or GBE, the concentrated form of the herb. *As a general memory booster and for poor circulation:* Take 120 mg of GBE daily, divided into two or three doses. *For Alzheimer's disease, depression, tinnitus, dizziness, impotence or other conditions caused by insufficient blood flow to the brain:* Take up to 240 mg a day.

GUIDELINES FOR USE: It commonly takes four to six weeks, and in some cases up to 12 weeks, for the herb's effects to be noticed. Generally, it is considered safe for long-term use in recommended dosages. You can take ginkgo with or without food. No adverse effects have been reported in pregnant or breastfeeding women who take the herb.

Possible side effects

In rare cases, ginkgo may cause irritability, restlessness, diarrhoea, nausea or vomiting, but these effects are usually mild and transient. People starting to take the herb may also notice headaches during the first day or two of use. If side effects are troublesome, discontinue ginkgo or reduce the dosage.

Ginseng

Panax ginseng
P. quinquefolius
Eleutherococcus senticosus

Common uses

- *Combats the physical effects of stress.*
- *Boosts vitality and enhances immunity.*
- *Chinese ginseng may treat impotence and infertility in men.*

Forms

- Capsule
- Dried herb/tea
- Powder
- Softgel
- Tablet
- Tincture

There are three main types of ginseng, any of which can exert a variety of protective effects on the body when taken at the correct dosage. Chinese ginseng is frequently added to manufactured beverages, but the amounts used are usually too small to be effective.

What it is

Panax ginseng – also called Asian, Chinese or Korean ginseng – has been used in Chinese medicine for thousands of years to enhance both longevity and the quality of life; it is the most widely available and extensively studied form of the herb. Another species, Panax quinquefolius, or American ginseng, is grown mainly in the American Midwest and exported to China. Siberian ginseng (Eleutherococcus senticosus) comes from Siberia, and is distantly related to the other two.

The medicinal part of the plant is its slow-growing root, which is harvested after four to six years, when its overall ginsenoside content – the main active ingredient in Panax ginsengs – is at its peak; there are 13 different ginsenosides in all. Panax ginsengs also contains panaxans, substances that can lower blood sugar, and polysaccharides, complex sugar molecules that enhance the immune system. 'White' ginseng is simply the dried root; 'red' ginseng (usually from Korea) has been steamed and dried. Most research studies have been done with white Chinese ginseng. Siberian ginseng is characterised by containing eleutherosides, which have similar properties to ginsenosides.

What it does

The primary health benefits of the three ginsengs derive from their antioxidant properties, their power to stimulate the immune system, and their ability to protect the body against the adverse effects of stress.

PREVENTION: All three ginsengs may help the body to combat a range of illnesses. They stimulate the production of specialised immune cells called 'killer T cells', which destroy harmful viruses and bacteria.

Research has also indicated that Chinese ginseng may inhibit the growth of certain cancer cells. A large Korean study found that the risk of cancer developing in people who took Panax ginseng was half that in subjects who did not take it. Although ginseng powders and tinctures

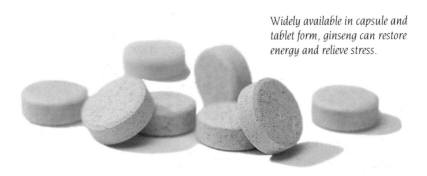

Widely available in capsule and tablet form, ginseng can restore energy and relieve stress.

were shown to lower the risk of cancer, eating fresh ginseng root or drinking ginseng juice or tea did not have the same effect.

ADDITIONAL BENEFITS: Ginseng may benefit people who are feeling fatigued and stressed and those recovering from long illnesses. It has been shown to balance the release of stress hormones in the body and to support the organs that produce these hormones: the pituitary gland and hypothalamus at the base of the brain, and the adrenal glands, located on top of the kidneys.

Chinese ginseng may help to correct impotence by improving erectile function through dilating blood vessels. Animal studies indicate that it increases testosterone levels and sperm production, bringing potential benefit to men with fertility problems.

Many long-distance runners and body-builders take ginseng to boost physical endurance. Herbalists believe that the ginsengs can combat fatigue by raising vitality. While Chinese ginseng is more applicable to the male system, Siberian ginseng may be more suitable for women, particularly those with menstrual cycle irregularities. American ginseng is highly regarded for its tonic effects, and has traditionally been used for treating digestive tract disorders. Otherwise the three ginsengs have many similarities in properties and use.

How to take it

DOSAGE: *For general health or to combat fatigue:* Take 100 to 250 mg *Panax ginseng* extract (or 300 to 400 mg Siberian ginseng) once or twice a day. *To support the body in times of stress or during recovery from illness:* Take the above dose twice a day. *For male impotence and infertility:* Take the above dose twice a day.

GUIDELINES FOR USE: Start at the lower end of the dosage range and increase your intake gradually. Some experts recommend that you stop taking ginseng for a week every two or three weeks and then resume your regular dose. In some cases, ginseng may be rotated with other herbs which stimulate the immune system, such as astragalus.

Possible side effects

At the recommended doses, ginseng is unlikely to cause any side effects. There have been reports that higher doses cause nervousness, insomnia, headache and stomach upset; if you have any of these problems, reduce your dose. The combination of ginseng and caffeine may intensify these reactions. Some women report increased menstrual bleeding or breast tenderness with high doses of Chinese ginseng. If this occurs, try using Siberian ginseng instead.

Glucosamine

This promising arthritis fighter helps to build cartilage – which provides cushioning at the tips of the bones – and protects and strengthens the joints as it relieves pain and stiffness. Although your body produces its own glucosamine, supplements can be helpful.

Common uses

- *Relieves pain, stiffness and swelling of the knees, fingers and other joints caused by osteoarthritis or rheumatoid arthritis.*
- *Helps to reduce arthritic back and neck pain.*
- *May speed up the healing of sprains and strengthen joints, preventing future injury.*

Forms

- Capsule
- Cream and skin patches
- Tablet

CAUTION!

REMINDER: If you have a medical condition, consult your doctor before taking supplements.

What it is

Glucosamine (pronounced glue-KOSE-a-mean) is a fairly simple molecule that contains the sugar glucose. It is found in relatively high concentrations in the joints and connective tissues, where the body uses it to form the larger molecules necessary for cartilage repair and maintenance. In recent years glucosamine has become available as a nutritional supplement. Various forms are sold, including glucosamine sulphate and N-acetyl-glucosamine (NAG). Glucosamine sulphate is the preferred form for arthritis: it is readily used by the body (90% to 98% is absorbed through the intestine) and appears to be very effective in relieving this condition.

What it does

Although some doctors hail glucosamine as an arthritis cure, no single supplement or combination of supplements can claim that title. Glucosamine does, however, provide significant relief from pain and inflammation for about half of arthritis sufferers – especially those with the common age-related form known as osteoarthritis. It can also help people with rheumatoid arthritis and other types of joint injuries.

✪ **MAJOR BENEFITS:** Used to treat arthritis in about 70 countries around the world, glucosamine can ease pain and inflammation, increase range of motion, and help to repair ageing and damaged joints in the knees, hips, spine and hands. Recent studies show that it may be even more effective for relieving pain and inflammation than nonsteroidal anti-inflammatory drugs (NSAIDs), such as aspirin and ibuprofen, commonly taken by arthritis sufferers – without their harmful side effects. Moreover, while NSAIDs mask arthritis pain, they do little to combat progression of the disease – and may even make it worse by impairing the body's ability to build cartilage. By contrast, glucosamine helps to make cartilage and may repair damaged joints. Although it cannot do much for people with advanced arthritis, when cartilage has completely worn away, it may benefit the millions of people with mild to moderately severe symptoms.

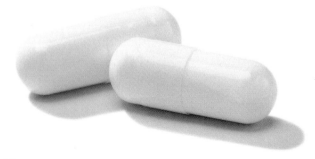

✱ **ADDITIONAL BENEFITS:** As a general joint strengthener, glucosamine may be useful for the prevention of arthritis and all forms of age-related degenerative joint disease. It may also speed healing of acute joint injuries, such as a sprained ankle or finger. Athletes and sportsmen and women often take glucosamine to help to prevent muscle injuries.

How to take it

▢ **DOSAGE:** The usual dosage for arthritis and other conditions is 500 mg glucosamine sulphate three times a day, or 1500 mg daily. This amount has been shown to be safe for all individuals and effective for most.

◉ **GUIDELINES FOR USE:** Glucosamine is typically taken long term and appears to be very safe. It may not bring relief as quickly as conventional pain relievers or anti-inflammatories do (it usually works in two to eight weeks), but its benefits are far greater and longer lasting when it is used over a period of time. Take glucosamine with meals to minimise the chance of digestive upset.

In addition to glucosamine, some supplements contain a related cartilage component called chondroitin sulphate and sometimes other nutrients, such as niacin or S-adenosylmethionine (SAM). These are purported to have enhanced cartilage-building properties, but research-based evidence for such benefits is lacking. Other supplements that are sometimes taken along with glucosamine for the relief of arthritis include boswellia, a tree extract from India; devil's claw from Namibia; celery seed extract; and the topical pain reliever cayenne cream. No adverse reactions have been reported when glucosamine is used with other supplements or with prescription or over-the-counter medications.

Possible side effects

Supplements of glucosamine – a natural substance produced in the body – appear to be virtually free of side effects, although no long-term studies have been done. Gastrointestinal effects, such as indigestion or nausea, are rare in those who take glucosamine supplements. Should any of these symptoms occur, try taking glucosamine with meals.

Goldenseal

Hydrastis canadensis

The Cherokee, Iroquois and other Native American tribes valued goldenseal as a remedy for everything from insect bites and bloating to eye infections and stomach aches. Today the root of this herb is used by medical herbalists in the USA and throughout Europe.

Common uses

- Soothes inflamed mucous membranes, as in sinusitis.
- Promotes healing of mouth ulcers and cold sores and helps to destroy the virus that causes warts.
- Bolsters the immune system.
- Alleviates digestive disorders.
- May help urinary tract infections.
- Treats eye infections.

Forms

- Capsule
- Dried herb/tea
- Liquid
- Ointment/cream
- Softgel
- Tincture

CAUTION!

- Goldenseal should not be used by pregnant women or people with high blood pressure or glaucoma.

REMINDER: *If you have a medical condition, consult your doctor before taking supplements.*

What it is

Related to the buttercup, goldenseal is a perennial herb native to North America. The dried root has long been used to soothe inflamed or infected mucous membranes; today it is appreciated for its ability to help the body to fight infection. The plant was first called goldenseal in the 19th century, acquiring its name from the rich yellow of the root and the small cuplike scars found there. These scars, which appear on the previous year's root growth, resemble the wax seals formerly used to close envelopes – hence the name 'goldenseal'.

The key medicinal compounds in goldenseal are the alkaloids berberine and hydrastine. Berberine is also responsible for the root's rich yellow colour – so vibrant, in fact, that Native Americans and early settlers utilised goldenseal as a dye as well as a medicinal herb. The alkaloids have a bitter taste, so goldenseal tea often includes other herbs or is mixed with a sweetener such as honey.

What it does

The primary benefit of goldenseal is its overall effect on immunity. Not only does it increase the power of the immune system to fight infection, but it can also combat both bacteria and viruses directly.

PREVENTION: Taking goldenseal as soon as you detect symptoms of a cold or flu may prevent the illness from developing fully – or at least minimise the symptoms – by enhancing the activity of virus-fighting white blood cells.

ADDITIONAL BENEFITS: Goldenseal fights bacteria, making it useful for mild urinary tract infections (if you begin taking it early enough) and

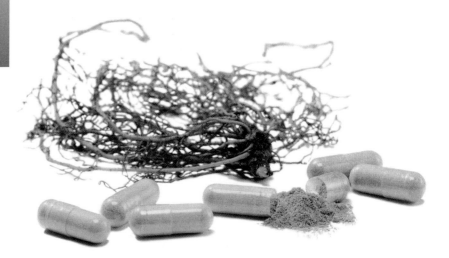

The root of the goldenseal plant is dried and then ground to a powder for use in supplements.

sinus infections. It may also help to soothe nausea and vomiting by stimulating digestive secretions and working to destroy the bacteria that may be causing the symptoms.

As one of several herbs that stimulate the immune system – others include echinacea, pau d'arco and astragalus – goldenseal can play a role in relieving the symptoms of chronic fatigue syndrome, a disabling disorder that may be partly caused by a weakened immune system. It also helps to fight cold sores and shingles (both caused by the herpes virus). Unless advised otherwise by a practitioner, use it for no more than a week or two at a time.

Applied topically, goldenseal tincture is beneficial for mouth ulcers and warts. The tincture promotes the healing of the sores and directly fights the human papilloma virus that causes warts. Once cooled and strained, goldenseal tea can be used as an eyewash to relieve eye infections such as conjunctivitis. Be sure to prepare a fresh batch daily, and store it in a sterile container so the tea does not get contaminated.

How to take it

🗒 **Dosage:** *For colds, flu and other respiratory infections:* As soon as you begin to feel symptoms, take 125 mg of goldenseal extract (in combination with 200 mg of echinacea extract) up to four times a day for no more than five days. *For urinary tract infections:* Drink several cups of goldenseal tea a day. *For nausea and vomiting:* Take 125 mg extract every four hours as needed. *For chronic fatigue syndrome:* Use 125 mg extract twice a day in rotation with other immune-stimulating herbs. *For cold sores and shingles:* Take 125 mg of goldenseal extract with 200 mg echinacea extract four times a day. *For mouth ulcers and warts:* Apply goldenseal tincture directly to the sores three times a day. *For eye infections:* Use 1 teaspoon dried herb per 600 ml of hot water. Steep, strain through muslin or a fine cloth and cool, then apply as an eyewash three times a day; make a new solution every day.

◉ **Guidelines for use:** Take goldenseal supplements with meals. Unlike echinacea and other herbs that stimulate the immune system, goldenseal should be used only when you feel that you are coming down with a cold, flu or some other illness, and only for the duration of the illness. The single exception to this rule is when you are taking goldenseal in rotation with other herbs to strengthen the immune system.

Possible side effects

When taken at recommended doses and for suggested lengths of time, goldenseal is safe to use and has few side effects. Very high doses may irritate the mucous membranes of the mouth and cause them to become excessively dry.

CASE HISTORY
Going for gold

Alexa K. always reacted badly to antibiotics. Although she needed them to combat her sinus infections, the side effects – dizziness, nausea, diarrhoea – often made the drugs worse than the illness.

When a herbalist told her to try goldenseal extract, Alexa was sceptical. But she took the goldenseal, and in a few days her sinus infection was gone – without a single side effect.

Now goldenseal is a part of Alexa's sinus first-aid kit. At the first sign of an infection she starts taking it, along with the immune stimulator echinacea.

Though antibiotics are sometimes necessary, in the past few years Alexa has often been able to avoid them. 'Those miserable side effects are history!' she reports.

Gotu kola

Centella asiatica

Common uses

- Treats burns and wounds.
- Builds connective tissue.
- Strengthens veins.
- Improves memory.

Forms

- Capsule
- Dried herb/tea
- Powder
- Tablet
- Tincture

CAUTION!

- **Pregnant women should not use gotu kola.**

REMINDER: If you have a medical condition, consult your doctor before taking supplements.

Reputed to be a favourite food of elephants, famously long-lived animals, gotu kola is associated by many people with longevity. Though scientific research has not shown that the herb can extend your life, there is little doubt that it provides important health benefits.

What it is

The medicinal use of gotu kola has its roots in India, where the herb continues to be part of the ancient healing tradition called Ayurveda. Word of its therapeutic benefits for skin disorders gradually spread throughout Asia and Europe, and in fact gotu kola has been used in France since the 1880s to treat burns and other wounds.

A red-flowered plant that thrives in hot, swampy areas, gotu kola grows naturally in India, Sri Lanka, Madagascar, middle and southern Africa, Australia, China and the southern USA. The appearance of this slender creeping perennial changes according to whether it is growing in water (broad, fan-shaped leaves) or on dry land (small, thin leaves). The plant's leaf is most commonly used medicinally.

What it does

Whether taken internally or applied externally as a compress, gotu kola has many beneficial effects. Components of the herb include chemicals called triterpenes (especially asiaticoside), which appear to enhance the formation of collagen in bones, cartilage and connective tissue. In addition they promote healthy blood vessels and may help to balance the activity of neurotransmitters, the chemical messengers in the brain.

MAJOR BENEFITS: Gotu kola's singular effect on connective tissue – promoting its healthy development and inhibiting the formation of hardened areas – makes it potentially important for treating many skin conditions. It can be therapeutic for burns, keloids (overgrown scar tissue) and wounds (including surgical incisions and skin ulcers). Gotu kola also seems to strengthen cells in the walls of blood vessels, improving blood flow, which makes it valuable in the treatment of varicose veins. Research results are often impressive. In more than a dozen studies observing gotu kola's effect on veins (which are surrounded by supportive connective-tissue sheaths), about 80% of patients with varicose veins and similar problems showed substantial improvement. Other studies indicate that applying gotu kola topically to psoriasis lesions may aid healing in sufferers of this condition as well.

ADDITIONAL BENEFITS: Gotu kola has been used to increase mental acuity for thousands of years. Current research supports a role for the herb in boosting memory, improving learning capabilities and possibly reversing some of the memory loss associated with Alzheimer's disease.

In one study, 30 children with learning difficulties were found to have significantly better concentration and attention levels after taking gotu kola for 12 weeks than they did at the start of the study. Early findings reveal that animals given gotu kola for two weeks were able to learn and remember new behaviours much better than animals not given the herb.

How to take it

⬜ **DOSAGE:** *To treat varicose veins*: Take 200 mg of the standardised extract three times a day. *For burns*: Use 200 mg twice a day until they heal. *To improve memory or possibly slow down the progress of Alzheimer's disease*: Take 200 mg three times a day. You can substitute 1 gram of the crude herb for each 200 mg dose of the standardised extract.

◉ **GUIDELINES FOR USE:** In most cases gotu kola is taken internally as a tablet or capsule, with or without meals, but gotu kola tea or tincture can also be applied externally to the skin for psoriasis, burns, wounds, incisions or scars. You can use both oral and topical preparations of the herb over the same period of time.

To apply gotu kola topically, soak a compress in tea or tincture and apply it directly to problem areas. Start with a relatively weak solution and increase the strength as needed. To brew gotu kola tea, steep 1 or 2 teaspoons of dried leaf in a cup of very hot water for 10 to 15 minutes. You can also make a paste to apply to patches of skin affected by psoriasis: break open capsules and mix 2 teaspoons of dried gotu kola powder in a small amount of water.

Possible side effects

Taking gotu kola orally or using a topical preparation generally does not cause problems. Skin rash (dermatitis), sensitivity to sunlight and headaches are rare side effects. If you experience these symptoms, reduce the dosage or stop using the herb.

FACTS & TIPS

▪ Gotu kola is also known as *Centella asiatica*, Indian pennywort, Indian water navelwort, talepetrako or hydrocotyle. Marsh penny-wort (*Hydrocotyle vulgaris*), a related species native to Europe, has no known therapeutic properties.

▪ Though the names sound similar, there is no relationship between gotu kola and the kola (or cola) nut used in cola drinks. The kola nut is a stimulant containing caffeine; gotu kola is a very mild sedative and is caffeine-free.

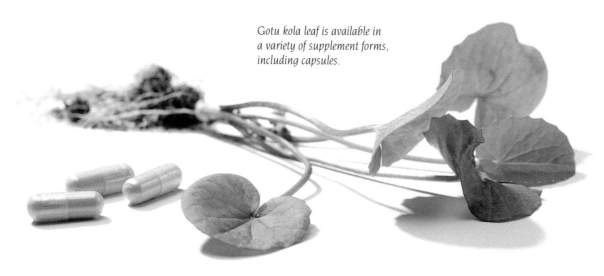

Gotu kola leaf is available in a variety of supplement forms, including capsules.

Grape seed extract

With antioxidant properties many times more powerful than vitamin C or vitamin E, grape seed extract can do much to promote a healthy heart and to reduce the risk of cancer. It also has the power to improve well-being in myriad ways.

Common uses

- *Treats blood vessel disorders.*
- *Protects against damage to vision.*
- *Lessens the risk of heart disease and cancer.*
- *Reduces the rate of collagen breakdown in the skin.*

Forms

- Capsule
- Liquid
- Tablet

What it is

An extract from the tiny seeds of red grapes has become one of the leading natural medicines in Europe. It belongs to the group of plant substances called flavonoids – antioxidants which protect the body's cells from damage by unstable oxygen molecules called free radicals. Grape seed extract contains oligomeric proanthocyanidin complexes (OPCs), also called proanthocyanidins. Once called pycnogenols (pik-NODGE-en-alls), OPCs are believed to play an important role in preventing heart disease and cancer. 'Pycnogenol' with a capital P is the trademark for a specific OPC derived from maritime pine bark; it can be used in place of grape seed extract, but it is more expensive, and many practitioners do not believe that it is worth the extra cost.

What it does

Grape seed extract exerts a powerful, positive influence on blood vessels. It is no coincidence that the active substances in this extract, OPCs, are key ingredients in one of the drugs most frequently prescribed for blood vessel (vascular) disorders in western Europe.

Grape seed extract contains both oil-soluble and water-soluble components, so it can penetrate all types of cell membranes, delivering antioxidant protection throughout the body. It is also one of the few substances that can cross the blood-brain barrier, which means that it may protect brain cells from free-radical damage.

✪ **MAJOR BENEFITS:** With its powerful ability to enhance the health of blood vessels, grape seed extract may not only reduce the risk of heart attack and stroke but also strengthen fragile or weak capillaries and increase blood flow, particularly to the extremities. For this reason many practitioners find it a beneficial supplement for almost any type

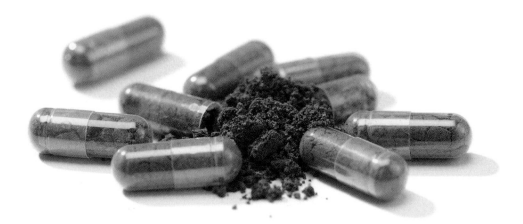

of vascular insufficiency as well as for conditions that are associated with poor vascular function, including diabetes, varicose veins, some cases of impotence, numbness and tingling in the arms and legs, and even painful leg cramps.

Grape seed extract affects even the tiniest blood vessels, so it can have a beneficial impact on circulation in the eye. It is often recommended as a supplement to combat macular degeneration and cataracts – two of the most common causes of blindness in elderly people. Grape seed extract may also be beneficial in people who regularly use computers. At least one study has shown that taking 300 mg of the extract daily for just 60 days reduced eye strain related to computer monitor work and improved contrast vision.

Many practitioners now endorse grape seed extract for its cancer-fighting properties. Working as antioxidants, OPCs correct damage to the genetic material of cells that could possibly cause tumours to form. ✱ **ADDITIONAL BENEFITS:** Grape seed extract helps to preserve and reinforce the collagen in the skin, so it is often included in cosmetic creams to improve skin elasticity.

Relief from allergy symptoms is another benefit of the extract; it inhibits the release of symptom-causing compounds such as histamine, which, in turn, helps to control a variety of allergic reactions, from hay fever to urticaria. The extract also blocks the release of prostaglandins, chemicals involved in allergic reactions and in pain and inflammation, particularly that of the menstrual disorder called endometriosis.

How to take it

🖉 **DOSAGE:** *For antioxidant protection*: Take 100 mg daily. *For therapeutic benefits*: Doses are usually 200 mg daily. Choose supplements that are standardised to contain 92% to 95% proanthocyanidins, or OPCs.
◈ **GUIDELINES FOR USE:** After 24 hours, only about 28% of grape seed extract's active components remain in the body, so it is important to take supplements at the same time every day, particularly when they are used to combat disease.

Possible side effects

No side effects from taking grape seed extract have been reported, and no toxic reactions have been noted.

Green tea

Camellia sinensis

According to Chinese legend, green tea was first drunk about 2700 BC, when an emperor sitting under a tea bush saw a few leaves fall into his cup of hot water – and sipped the brew. This type of tea has now been discovered to contain a highly promising anticancer compound.

Common uses
- May help to prevent cancer.
- Protects against heart disease.
- Inhibits tooth decay.
- Promotes longevity.

Forms
- Capsule
- Liquid
- Powder
- Tablet
- Tea

CAUTION!

- Pregnant and breastfeeding women should limit their consumption of green tea to two cups a day.

REMINDER: *If you have a medical condition, consult your doctor before taking supplements.*

What it is

The traditional process that yields green tea is simple: the leaves from the tea plant are first steamed, then rolled and dried. The steaming kills enzymes that would otherwise ferment the leaves. With other types of tea the leaves are allowed to ferment either partially (for oolong tea) or fully (for black tea). The lack of fermentation gives green tea its unique flavour and, more importantly, preserves virtually all the naturally present polyphenols – strong antioxidants that can protect against cell damage. Other substances in green tea that may also be beneficial are fluoride, catechins and tannins.

What it does

Green tea possesses compounds that may provide powerful protection against several cancers and, possibly, heart disease. Studies indicate that it also fights infection and promotes longevity.

PREVENTION: The prevalence of certain types of cancer is lower among people who drink green tea. In one large-scale study researchers found that Chinese men and women who drank green tea as seldom as once a week for six months had lower rates of rectal, pancreatic and possibly colon cancers than those who rarely or never drank it. In women, the risk of rectal or pancreatic cancer was nearly halved. Preliminary research suggests that green tea may also provide protection against breast, stomach and skin cancers.

Studies investigating how green tea might guard against cancer have pointed to the potency of its main antioxidant, the polyphenol EGCG (epigallocatechin-gallate). Some scientists believe that EGCG may be one of the most effective anticancer compounds ever discovered, protecting cells from damage and boosting the body's own production of antioxidant enzymes. One US study found that EGCG prompts cancer cells to stop reproducing by stimulating a natural process of programmed cell death called apoptosis. Remarkably, EGCG does not cause damage to healthy cells. Separate research at the Medical College of Ohio indicates that EGCG inhibits the production of urokinase, an enzyme that cancer cells need in order to grow. In animals, blocking urokinase shrinks tumours and sometimes causes the cancer to go into complete remission.

ADDITIONAL BENEFITS: The antioxidant effect of the polyphenols in green tea may also help to protect the heart. In test-tube studies these compounds appeared to suppress the damage to LDL cholesterol, thought to be an initial step in the build-up of plaque in the arteries. A Japanese study of 1371 men linked daily consumption of green tea to the prevention of heart disease. In addition, green tea contains fluoride, which provides an overall antibacterial effect and may help to guard against tooth decay. Preliminary evidence suggests that green tea may also have a beneficial effect on arthritis and in the healing of wounds.

How to take it

 DOSAGE: You can get the benefits of green tea either by taking green tea capsules or tablets, or by drinking several cups of the brew each day. Your aim should be to take in 240 to 320 mg of polyphenols.

When using supplements, buy those standardised to contain at least 50% polyphenols. At this concentration two 250 mg supplements would provide 250 mg of polyphenols. Studies show that four cups of freshly brewed green tea also supply a recommended amount of polyphenols.

 GUIDELINES FOR USE: Take green tea supplements at meals with a full glass of water. Drink freshly brewed green tea either on its own or with meals. To make tea, use 1 teaspoon of green tea leaves per 225 ml of very hot water. Let the brew steep for three to five minutes; then strain and drink it.

Possible side effects

Green tea is very safe both as a supplement and as a beverage, but people who are sensitive to caffeine may not want to drink large amounts of it because each cup contains about 40 mg of caffeine. Green tea supplements, however, have very little caffeine. The recommended dose of green tea supplements provides the same amount of polyphenols as four cups of green tea, but generally contains only 5 to 6 mg of caffeine.

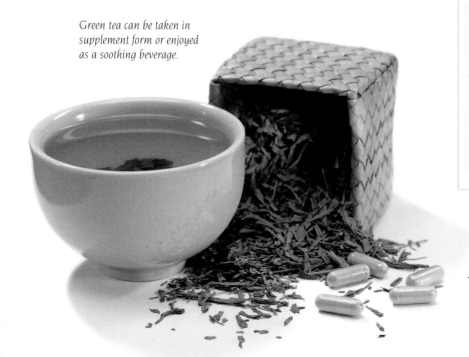

Green tea can be taken in supplement form or enjoyed as a soothing beverage.

Hawthorn

Crataegus oxyacantha

If you are diagnosed with any form of heart disease you will want to know all about hawthorn. This herb, historically used both as a diuretic and as a treatment for kidney and bladder stones, is now one of the most widely prescribed remedies for heart problems.

Common uses

- Relieves the chest pain of angina.
- Lowers high blood pressure.
- Helps the heart to pump more efficiently in people with heart disease.
- Corrects irregular heartbeat (cardiac arrhythmia).

Forms

- Capsule
- Dried herb/tea
- Powder
- Tablet
- Tincture

CAUTION!

REMINDER: If you have a medical condition, consult your doctor before taking supplements.

What it is

For centuries hawthorn, a shrub or tree that grows up to 9 metres high, has been trimmed to hedge height and planted along the edges of fields or as a garden boundary. As a divider it both looks attractive and discourages trespassers: it produces pretty white flowers and vibrant red berries, but it also has large thorns. (The crown of thorns worn by Christ at the Crucifixion is believed to have been woven from hawthorn twigs.)

Knowledge of the cardioprotective benefits of hawthorn was widespread among peoples of different eras and locations, from the ancient Greeks to the Native Americans, who considered the herb a potent heart tonic. Modern use of hawthorn originated with the 19th-century Irish physician Dr D. Greene of Ennis, who had great success in treating heart disease. Greene guarded his heart formula closely, and it was not until after his death in the 1890s that his secret remedy was revealed to be tincture of hawthorn berry.

What it does

Hawthorn is a herb that directly benefits the workings of the heart and the arteries. It can dilate blood vessels, increase the heart's energy supply and improve its pumping ability. These gentle but valuable cardiac effects can probably be traced to its abundant supply of plant compounds called flavonoids – especially oligomeric proanthocyanidin complexes (OPCs) – which function as potent antioxidants.

Hawthorn supplements are derived from the plant's leaves and flowers, its red berries (right), or a combination of all three.

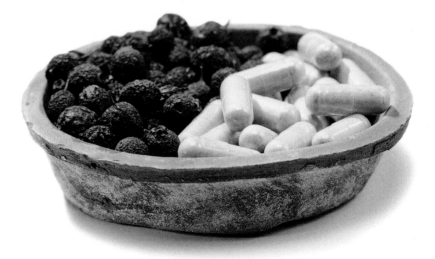

⊠ **MAJOR BENEFITS:** Hawthorn can have beneficial effects on the heart. It widens the arteries by interfering with an enzyme called ACE (angiotensin-converting enzyme), which constricts blood vessels. This action improves blood flow through the arteries, which makes the herb a good remedy for people with angina. In addition, chronically constricted arteries can lead to high blood pressure (because the heart must work harder to pump blood through inflexible arteries), so hawthorn may reduce blood pressure in those with mild hypertension.

Hawthorn also seems to block enzymes that weaken the heart muscle, thereby strengthening its pumping power. This property makes it especially useful for people with mild heart disease who do not need strong heart medications such as digitalis. Moreover, the antioxidant properties of hawthorn may help to protect against damage associated with the build-up of plaque in the coronary arteries.

⊠ **ADDITIONAL BENEFITS:** Hawthorn has a long history as a treatment for other conditions as well. It seems to exert a calming effect and functions as a sleeping aid in some people who suffer from insomnia. Several researchers have also noted that hawthorn preserves collagen – the protein that composes connective tissue – which is damaged in such diseases as arthritis.

How to take it

⊘ **DOSAGE:** The recommended dose of hawthorn extract ranges from 300 to 450 mg a day in capsule or tablet form, and from 1 teaspoon to 1 tablespoon of the tincture, depending on the type of heart condition. People at risk of heart disease may wish to take a 100 to 150 mg supplement or 1 teaspoon of the tincture daily as a heart disease preventative.

◉ **GUIDELINES FOR USE:** If you are taking large doses, hawthorn works best when the daily amount is split up and taken at three different times during the day. Hawthorn may take a couple of months to build up in your system and produce noticeable results.

Possible side effects

Hawthorn is widely regarded as one of the safest herbal preparations. Although there have been reports of nausea, sweating, fatigue and skin rashes, these side effects are rare. Hawthorn appears to be safe to use with drugs prescribed for heart disease; you may even need less of some heart medications while you are taking it. But consult your doctor before trying hawthorn, and never stop taking a prescribed drug (or reduce the dose) except on your doctor's advice.

RECENT FINDINGS

In an eight-week German study of 136 people with mild to moderate heart disease, those taking hawthorn extract reported less shortness of breath, less ankle swelling, and better exercise performance than those given a placebo. Physical examinations and laboratory tests confirmed that the condition of the hawthorn group improved, while the condition of the placebo group worsened.

DID YOU KNOW?

In ancient lore, hawthorn was said to protect houses from lightning, and to protect people from the evil spirits that roamed the Earth on the eve of festivals such as May Day, but it was bad luck to take its blossom indoors.

Iodine

Many people associate iodine with the orange-brown topical antiseptic used to clean childhood cuts and grazes, but the real value of this potent trace mineral springs from its role in the manufacture of thyroxine, the hormone responsible for regulating metabolism.

Common uses

- *Corrects an iodine deficiency.*
- *Ensures proper functioning of the thyroid gland.*
- *May help to treat fibrocystic breasts.*

Forms

- Capsule
- Liquid
- Tablet

What it is

Although the body needs only tiny amounts of iodine, this mineral is so crucial to an individual's overall health that in the 1920s US government officials decided that it should be added to a foodstuff common to nearly everyone – table salt. The introduction of iodised salt to the American diet virtually eliminated one severe form of mental retardation called cretinism. In the UK salt is not routinely iodised, although you can buy an iodised brand of salt if you wish to supplement iodine in this way. Apart from iodised salt, fish and seafood are the best dietary sources of iodine, as well as fruit, vegetables and cereals grown in iodine-rich soil.

Despite the recognised importance of this vital mineral, however, about 1.6 billion people in the world, mostly in developing countries, still suffer from iodine deficiency.

What it does

Unique among minerals, iodine has only one known function in the body: it is essential to the thyroid gland for manufacturing thyroxine, a hormone that regulates metabolism in all the body's cells.

PREVENTION: By getting enough iodine, a pregnant woman can prevent certain types of mental retardation in her developing foetus.

ADDITIONAL BENEFITS: Unlike many other minerals, iodine does not seem to help in the treatment of specific diseases, but it plays a crucial role in assuring the health of the thyroid, the butterfly-shaped gland that surrounds the windpipe (trachea). When your iodine intake is adequate your body contains about 40 mg of it, and 75% of that amount is stored in the thyroid. This gland controls the body's overall metabolism, which determines how quickly and efficiently calories are burned. It also regulates growth and development in children, reproduction, nerve and muscle function, the breakdown of proteins and fats, the growth of nails

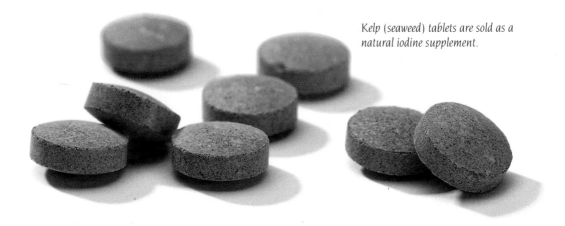

Kelp (seaweed) tablets are sold as a natural iodine supplement.

and hair, and the use of oxygen by every cell in the body. There is some evidence that iodine derived from an organic source may be effective in reducing the pain of fibrocystic breasts, but patients should discuss this type of supplementation with their doctor first.

How much you need

The recommended target for iodine is 140 mcg daily for adult men and women. One teaspoon of iodised salt contains about 300 mcg of iodine, but there is a wide range of other dietary sources (see below).

⊟ **IF YOU GET TOO LITTLE:** Iodine deficiency is extremely rare in developed countries, but the first signs include an enlarged thyroid gland, known as a goitre. Lack of iodine can cause the gland to expand in an attempt to increase its surface area and trap as much of the iodine in the bloodstream as possible. Although a low iodine intake can result in low levels of thyroid hormone (hypothyroidism), the most likely cause is a condition known as myxoedema, which results from autoimmune damage (when the body's immune system turns on itself). Hypothyroidism is characterised by fatigue, dry skin, a rise in blood fats, a hoarse voice, delayed reflexes and reduced mental clarity. Consult your doctor if you have these symptoms.

⊕ **IF YOU GET TOO MUCH:** There is very little risk of iodine overdose, even at levels 10 to 20 times the recommended amount. However, if you ingest 30 times the recommended amount you are likely to experience a metallic taste, mouth sores, swollen salivary glands, diarrhoea, vomiting, headache, a rash and difficulty in breathing. Ironically, a goitre can also develop if you consistently take extremely large amounts of iodine, which is one of the causes of thyrotoxicosis. This condition may be associated with high levels of thyroid hormone, leading to over-activity, rapid reflexes, anxiety and excessive weight loss.

How to take it

⊘ **DOSAGE:** You probably get all the iodine you need from your daily diet, especially if you regularly eat fish. Iodine is also a standard ingredient in many multivitamin and mineral supplements. People on a thyroid hormone should always discuss their condition with their doctor before taking individual iodine supplements.

◉ **GUIDELINES FOR USE:** When prescribed, iodine supplements can be taken at any time of the day, with or without food.

Other sources

The mineral can also be found in saltwater fish and in sea vegetation, such as kelp. Soil in coastal areas also tends to be iodine-rich, as are the dairy products derived from cows grazing there. The same is true for fruits and vegetables grown in soil high in iodine. Commercial baked goods – such as breads and cakes – can also be good sources of iodine.

Iron

A surprising number of people have insufficient iron in their diets – and few realise that lack of the mineral can make them weak, unable to concentrate and more susceptible than normal to infection. Too much iron, however, can be dangerous, so be cautious about taking supplements.

Common uses

- Treats iron-deficiency anaemia.
- Often needed during pregnancy; by women with heavy menstrual periods; or in other situations determined by your doctor.

Forms

- Capsule
- Liquid
- Softgel
- Tablet

CAUTION!

- Avoid high-dose supplements containing iron alone, unless they have been prescribed by your doctor. Some people suffer from haemochromatosis, an inherited disease which causes them to absorb too much iron, and most don't even know they have it. (Early symptoms include fatigue and aching joints.)

- A supplement containing iron alone could also mask a cause of anaemia, such as a bleeding ulcer, and prevent your doctor from making an early, life-saving diagnosis.

REMINDER: If you have a medical condition, consult your doctor before taking supplements.

What it is

Needed throughout the body, iron is an essential part of haemoglobin, the oxygen-carrying component of red blood cells. The mineral is also found in myoglobin, which supplies oxygen to the muscles, and is part of many enzymes and immune-system compounds. The body, which gets most of the iron it needs from foods, carefully monitors its iron status, absorbing more of the mineral when demand is high (during periods of rapid growth, such as pregnancy or childhood) and less when stores of it are adequate. Because the body loses iron when bleeding, menstruating women may often have low levels. Vegetarians, people on weight-loss diets and endurance athletes may experience iron shortfalls as well.

What it does

By helping the blood and muscles to deliver oxygen, iron supplies energy to every cell in the body. Yet iron deficiency is surprisingly common in the UK. According to government surveys, the majority of women do not reach their dietary target of 14.8 mg daily. Although for most people it is very difficult to develop an iron deficiency from poor nutrition (iron is found in many foods), women with heavy menstrual periods may be particularly at risk and will benefit from iron supplementation, as will people with medical conditions that give rise to iron-deficiency anaemia.

✪ **MAJOR BENEFITS:** Keeping your body well supplied with iron provides vitality, helps your immune system function at its best and gives your mind an edge. Studies show that even mild iron deficiency – well short of the levels commonly associated with anaemia – can cause adults to have a short attention span and teenagers to do poorly in school.

How much you need

The recommended daily amount for iron is 8.7 mg a day for men and for postmenopausal women. For younger women it is 14.8 mg a day, with no recommendation for an additional requirement during pregnancy. To combat anaemia, additional iron – through either diet or supplements – is typically needed for a period of weeks or months.

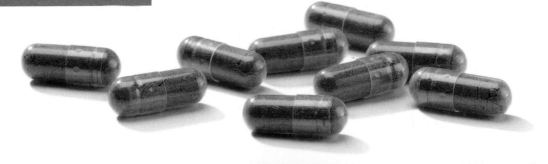

⊟ IF YOU GET TOO LITTLE: If you get too little iron in your diet or lose too much through heavy menstrual periods, stomach bleeding (commonly caused by arthritis drugs) or cancer, your body draws on its iron reserve. Initially there are no symptoms, but as your iron supply dwindles, so does your body's ability to produce healthy red blood cells. The result is iron-deficiency anaemia, marked by weakness, fatigue, paleness, breathlessness, palpitations and increased susceptibility to infection.

⊞ IF YOU GET TOO MUCH: Some studies link too much iron to an increased risk of chronic diseases, including heart disease and colon cancer. Excess iron can be particularly dangerous in adults with a genetic tendency to overabsorb it (haemochromatosis), and in children, who are especially susceptible to iron overdose.

How to take it

⊘ DOSAGE: Unless a practitioner advises otherwise, iron should be taken only in the form of a multivitamin or multimineral supplement at no more than the recommended daily amount. Anaemia requires a careful diagnosis, and treatment to correct the underlying cause. When prescribed by a doctor, iron is typically taken in a form called ferrous salts – usually ferrous sulphate, ferrous fumarate or ferrous gluconate. A typical prescribed dose provides about 30 mg of iron one to three times daily. Most men and postmenopausal women do not need iron supplements and should consider taking a multivitamin or multimineral supplement that does not contain this nutrient.

◉ GUIDELINES FOR USE: Iron is best absorbed when taken on an empty stomach. However, if iron upsets your stomach, have it with meals, preferably with a small amount of meat and a food or drink rich in vitamin C, such as broccoli or orange juice, to help boost the amount of iron your body absorbs.

Other sources

Iron-rich foods include liver, beef and lamb. Clams, oysters and mussels also contain iron. Vegetarians can get adequate amounts of iron from beans and peas, leafy green vegetables, dried fruits, such as apricots and raisins, and fortified breakfast cereals. Brewer's yeast, kelp, molasses and wheat bran are also good sources.

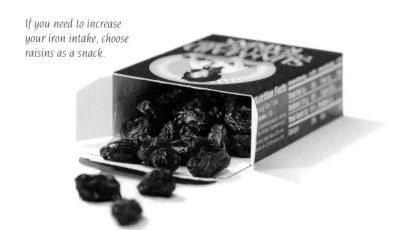

If you need to increase your iron intake, choose raisins as a snack.

Kelp and spirulina

Health enthusiasts are looking to the seas and lakes for algae and plant proteins that are powerful food supplements. Predominant among the aquatic plants that have been found to contain various beneficial substances are kelp and spirulina.

Common uses

Kelp
- *Treats an underactive thyroid gland.*
- *Provides essential nutrients.*

Spirulina
- *Treats bad breath.*
- *Adds protein, vitamins and minerals to the diet.*

Forms
- Capsule
- Liquid
- Powder
- Tablet
- Tincture

What they are

Kelp and spirulina are two very different types of aquatic alga. Kelp, a long-stemmed seaweed, is derived from various species of brown algae known as *Fucus* or *Laminaria*. It is a prime source of iodine, a mineral crucial in preventing thyroid problems.

The smaller spirulina (also known as a blue-green alga) is actually a single-celled microorganism, or microalga, that closely resembles a bacterium. Because its spiral-shaped filaments are rich in the plant pigment chlorophyll, spirulina turns the lakes and ponds where it grows a dark blue-green.

What they do

Kelp and spirulina have been used medicinally for thousands of years in China. Devotees make many claims for their powers – ranging from increased libido to reduced hair loss – but most are highly speculative. The algae do, however, have some confirmed medicinal properties.

✪ **MAJOR BENEFITS:** The high iodine content of kelp makes it useful for treating an underactive thyroid caused by a shortage of iodine. This remedy is rarely necessary, however, because iodised salt supplies plenty of this mineral. Kelp is also marketed as a weight-loss aid, but it is probably effective only in the extremely rare cases when weight gain is secondary to an iodine-deficient underactive thyroid. Kelp should be taken only under a doctor's close supervision for the treatment of thyroid disorders.

Spirulina is a prime source of chlorophyll so it is ideal for combating one of life's most troublesome minor complaints: bad breath. It can be an extremely effective remedy, provided that the condition is not due to gum disease or chronic sinusitis. Spirulina is a key ingredient of many commercial chlorophyll breath-fresheners.

Spirulina is the most popular of the blue-green algae supplements.

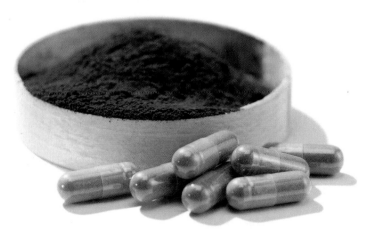

✱ **ADDITIONAL BENEFITS:** Sometimes kelp and spirulina are included in vegetarian and macrobiotic diets. In addition to iodine, kelp provides carotenoids as well as fatty acids, potassium, magnesium, calcium, iron and other nutrients. Spirulina contains protein, vitamins (including B_{12} and folic acid), carotenoids and other nutrients. The concentrations of all these substances appear to be fairly low, however. There are many less expensive – and better tasting – sources of vitamins and minerals than kelp and spirulina, including an array of popular garden vegetables.

Various other claims are made for kelp and spirulina – that they boost energy, relieve arthritis, enhance liver function, prevent heart disease and certain types of cancer, boost immunity, suppress HIV and AIDS, and protect cells against damage from X-rays or heavy metals such as lead. But most studies on these supplements have been done in test tubes or with animals, and more research is needed.

How to take them

▣ **DOSAGE:** *To use kelp for an underactive thyroid:* Use kelp only when it is recommended by your doctor; if iodine is needed, your doctor can prescribe an appropriate dose. Powder forms dissolve easily in water, though some people do not like the taste. Tablets, capsules and tinctures are equally effective.

To freshen the breath with spirulina: Use a commercial, chlorophyll-rich 'green' drink (the label will often say if the chlorophyll is derived in part from spirulina) or mix a teaspoon of spirulina powder in half a glass of water. Swish the liquid around the mouth, then swallow it. Alternatively, chew a tablet thoroughly and then swallow it. Repeat three or four times a day, or as needed.

◉ **GUIDELINES FOR USE:** Take with food to minimise the chances of digestive upset. Pregnant or breastfeeding women may want to avoid kelp because of its high iodine content, though spirulina seems to be very safe.

Possible side effects

Occasionally nausea or diarrhoea develops in those taking kelp or spirulina; if this side effect occurs, lower or stop the dose. Up to 3% of the population is sensitive to iodine and may experience adverse reactions to long-term ingestion of kelp – including a painful enlargement of the thyroid gland that disappears once the kelp is discontinued. This condition is most common in Japan, where seaweed is a dietary staple.

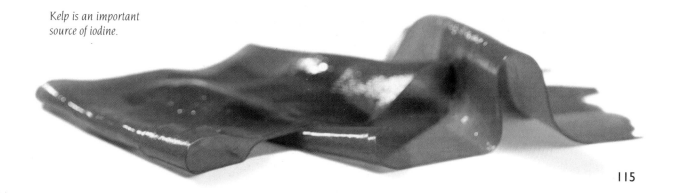

Kelp is an important source of iodine.

Lecithin and choline

These closely related nutrients with rather daunting scientific names are essential for the proper functioning of every cell in the body. They have particularly important roles to play in maintaining a healthy liver and nervous system.

Common uses

- Aid in the prevention of gallstones.
- Strengthen the liver, which makes them useful in the treatment of hepatitis and cirrhosis.
- Help the liver to eliminate toxins from the bodies of cancer patients undergoing chemotherapy.
- Diminish indigestion symptoms.
- May boost memory and enhance brain function.

Forms

- Capsule
- Liquid
- Powder
- Softgel
- Tablet

What they are

Lecithin (pronounced LESS-i-thin) is a fatty substance found in many animal and plant-based foods, including liver, eggs, soya beans, peanuts and wheat germ. It is often added to processed foods – including ice cream, chocolate, margarine and salad dressings – to help blend, or emulsify, the fats with water. It is also manufactured in the body.

Lecithin is considered an excellent source of choline, one of the B vitamins, primarily in the form called phosphatidylcholine. Once in the body, the phosphatidylcholine breaks down into choline, so that when you take lecithin, or absorb lecithin from foods, your body gets choline. However, only 10% to 20% of the lecithin found in plants and other natural sources consists of phosphatidylcholine.

Although dietary lecithin is a primary source of choline, choline is also found in liver, soya beans, egg yolks, grape juice, peanuts, cabbage and cauliflower. Choline supplements are available in health-food shops, and choline is a common ingredient of B-complex vitamins or other combination formulas.

What they do

Lecithin and choline are needed for a range of bodily functions. They help to build cell membranes and facilitate the movement of fats and nutrients in and out of cells. They aid in reproduction and in foetal and infant development; they are essential to liver and gall bladder health; and they may promote a healthy heart. Choline is also a key component of the brain chemical acetylcholine, which plays a prominent role in memory and muscle control.

As a result of their widely distributed effects, lecithin and choline have been touted for almost everything – from curing cancer and AIDS to lowering cholesterol. Even though the evidence for some of these claims is weak, the nutrients should not be dismissed out of hand.

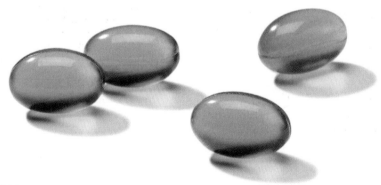

Lecithin supplements come in a variety of forms, including softgels.

✦ MAJOR BENEFITS: Lecithin and choline may be especially helpful in the treatment of gall bladder and liver diseases. Lecithin is a key component of bile, the fat-digesting substance, and low levels of this nutrient are known to precipitate gallstones. Taking supplements with lecithin or phosphatidylcholine, its purified extract, may help to treat or prevent this disorder. Lecithin may also be beneficial for the liver: the results of a ten-year study on baboons showed that it prevented severe liver scarring and cirrhosis caused by alcohol abuse, and other studies have indicated that it helps to relieve liver problems associated with hepatitis.

Choline is often included in liver complex formulas along with other liver-strengthening supplements, such as the amino acid methionine, the B vitamin inositol and the herbs milk thistle and dandelion. These preparations, sometimes called lipotropic combinations or factors, can protect against the build-up of fats within the liver, improve the flow of fats and cholesterol through the liver and gall bladder, and help the liver to rid the body of dangerous toxins. They may be especially effective in treating liver or gall bladder diseases, such as hepatitis, cirrhosis or gallstones, as well as conditions that benefit from good liver function, such as endometriosis (the leading cause of female infertility), and side effects from chemotherapy. Choline, along with the B vitamins pantothenic acid and thiamin, may also relieve indigestion.

✦ ADDITIONAL BENEFITS: These two nerve-building nutrients may be useful for improving memory in people with Alzheimer's disease, as well as for preventing neural tube birth defects (spina bifida), boosting performance in endurance sports and treating twitches and tics (tardive dyskinesia) caused by antipsychotic drugs. Lecithin and choline have also been proposed as possible remedies for high cholesterol and even cancer. However, more studies are needed to define their role in these and other diseases.

How to take them

✐ DOSAGE: Lecithin is usually given in a dosage of two 1200 mg capsules twice a day. It can also be taken in a granular form: 1 teaspoon contains 1200 mg of lecithin. Choline can be obtained from lecithin, although phosphatidylcholine (500 mg three times a day) or plain choline (500 mg three times a day) may be a better source. Choline can also be taken as part of a lipotropic combination product. In the UK no recommended amounts have been set for lecithin and choline, but the US Food and Drug Administration (FDA) has recognised choline as an essential nutrient and has recommended daily intakes of 550 mg for men and 425 mg for women.

✦ GUIDELINES FOR USE: Lecithin and choline should be taken with meals to enhance absorption. Granular lecithin has a nutty taste and can be sprinkled over foods or mixed into drinks.

Possible side effects

In high doses, lecithin and choline may cause sweating, nausea, vomiting, bloating and diarrhoea. Taking very high dosages of choline (10 grams a day) may produce a fishy body odour or a heart rhythm disorder.

Lutein

Lutein is a yellow pigment found in egg yolk, some algae, many plants and in the light sensitive cells at the back of the eye, where it helps to maintain healthy vision. Increased intake of lutein is linked with reduced risk of macular degeneration, the main cause of blindness in older people.

Common uses

- *Important for eye health.*
- *Essential for the development of the macular pigment which protects light sensitive cells in the retina from free radical dmage.*
- *May lower the risk of macular degeneration.*
- *May improve vision in people with cataracts.*
- *May provide protection against some cancers.*

Forms

- Capsule
- Softgel
- Sublingual spray
- Tablet

What it is

Lutein (and its chemical isomer zeaxanthin) is a member of the carotenoid family, *see page* 48. It gives the yellow colour to fruits and vegetables, such as mango, papaya, sweetcorn and tomato. However, the highest amounts of lutein are found in dark green vegetables such as kale, spinach and turnip greens. Broccoli, Brussels sprouts, peas, leeks and some types of lettuce, particularly Cos and Romaine lettuce are also good dietary sources. The greener the vegetable, the more lutein it contains, and raw vegetables are better sources than cooked.

The amount of lutein found in the average UK diet is between 1 mg and 3 mg a day. Though official UK recommendations for lutein intake have not been made, results of research suggest that an appropriate intake could be 6 mg a day. Even people who eat large quantities of fruit and vegetables could find that hard to manage.

What it does

Lutein is an antioxidant. This means that it has the ability to neutralise harmful free radicals (substances produced by pollution, radiation, fried and burnt foods, sunlight and combustion) that may have entered the body. These free radicals can damage cells and accelerate ageing. At one time, it was thought that all antioxidants served the same purpose but there is growing evidence that they have specific functions.

Lutein is thought to play an important role in maintaining healthy vision because it is the main pigment found in the central region of the retina, known as the macula. This is the region of maximum visual sensitivity. As we get older, the cells with retinal pigment become less efficient, the retina degenerates and central vision is gradually lost. This process is known as age-related macular degeneration (ARMD).

One of the causes of macular degeneration is damage from the free radicals in sunlight. Lutein may protect the macula by acting as an optical filter for sunlight and as an antioxidant to soak up the free radicals. Lutein may also play a role in maintaining immunity.

MAJOR BENEFITS: Scientific studies have generally found an increased risk of macular degeneration with low levels of lutein in the diet or in the blood; however, conclusive evidence that increased intakes will reduce the incidence of ARMD or help to treat it is not yet available. Small studies have provided encouraging results. A recent US study found that supplementation with lutein and other antioxidants in people with early ARMD had a beneficial effect on macular function. And another trial published in *Optometry* found that a daily dose of 10 mg lutein, alone or with other antioxidant supplements, improved visual function in 90 patients with atrophic ARMD over a period of 12 months.

Research looking at the role of lutein in cataract prevention has so far not been encouraging. But lutein supplements have been found to improve visual acuity and glare sensitivity in people with cataracts.

Pending the results of further research, it is important to consume a diet rich in leafy green vegetables, which should supply high amounts of lutein. If you do not like fresh vegetables, your diet may be lacking in this nutrient.

ADDITIONAL BENEFITS: High dietary intake of lutein has been linked with reduced risk of some cancers, most notably endometrial, ovarian and breast cancer. A US study found an intake of more than 7,300 mcg (7.3 mg) a day of lutein was associated with a 70 per cent reduced risk of endometrial cancer. The risk of ovarian cancer has been shown to be reduced by 40 per cent in women with a weekly intake of lutein of more than 24,000 mcg (24 mg) compared with a weekly intake of less than 3,800 mcg (3.8 mg). In another study, lutein intake of more than 7,162 mcg (7.162 mg) daily was associated with a 53 per cent reduction in the risk of developing breast cancer compared with consumption of less than 3652 mcg (3.652 mg) daily.

How to take it

DOSAGE: *For general good eye health*: Take 6 mg daily (if your diet does not contain dark leafy green vegetables.) Supplements containing these amounts are available. *For prevention*: To reduce the risk of eye disorders such as cataracts and macular degeneration, take 6-15 mg lutein daily.

GUIDELINES FOR USE: Take with food in a single daily dose. Benefits develop slowly and may not fully develop for six months to two years.

Possible side effects

There are no known side effects from either short-term or long-term use of lutein. No interactions with drugs have been found.

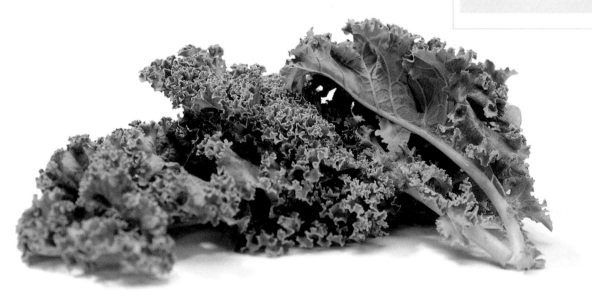

Magnesium

Although little heralded, magnesium may be one of the most important health-promoting minerals. Studies suggest that, as well as enhancing some 300 enzyme-related processes in the body, magnesium may help to prevent or combat many chronic diseases.

Common uses

- *Helps to protect against heart disease and arrhythmia.*
- *Eases symptoms of chronic fatigue and fibromyalgia.*
- *Lowers high blood pressure.*
- *May reduce the severity of asthma attacks.*
- *Improves symptoms of premenstrual syndrome (PMS).*
- *Aids in preventing the complications of diabetes.*

Forms

- Capsule
- Powder
- Tablet

CAUTION!

- People with kidney disease should seek medical advice before taking magnesium.

- Magnesium can reduce the effectiveness of tetracycline antibiotics.

REMINDER: *If you have a medical condition, consult your doctor before taking supplements.*

What it is

The average person's body contains just under 30 grams of magnesium, but this small amount is vital to a number of bodily functions. Many people do not have adequate stores of magnesium, often because they rely too heavily on processed foods, which contain very little of this mineral. In addition, magnesium levels are easily depleted by stress, certain diseases or medications and intense physical activity. For this reason, nutritional supplements may be needed for the maintenance of optimal health. Supplements come in many forms, including magnesium acetate, magnesium carbonate, magnesium citrate, magnesium gluconate, magnesium oxide and magnesium sulphate.

What it does

One of the most versatile minerals, magnesium is involved in energy production, nerve function, muscle relaxation and bone and tooth formation. In conjunction with calcium and potassium, magnesium regulates heart rhythm and clots blood; it also aids in the production and use of insulin.

PREVENTION: Recent research indicates that magnesium is beneficial for the prevention and treatment of heart disease. Studies show that the risk of dying of a heart attack is lower in areas with 'hard' water, which contains high levels of magnesium. Some researchers speculate that if everyone drank hard water the number of deaths from heart attacks might decline by 19%. Magnesium appears to lower blood pressure, and has also been found to aid recovery after a heart attack by inhibiting blood clots, widening arteries and normalising dangerous arrhythmias.

Preliminary studies suggest that an adequate intake of magnesium may help to prevent non-insulin-dependent (type 2) diabetes. American researchers at Johns Hopkins University measured magnesium levels in more than 12,000 people who did not have diabetes, then tracked them for six years to see who developed the disease. Individuals with the lowest magnesium levels had a 94% greater chance of developing the disease than those with the highest levels. Further studies are needed to see if magnesium supplements can prevent the disease.

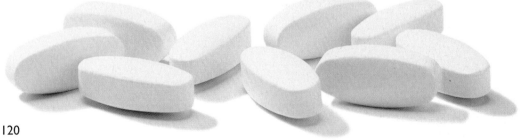

✛ **ADDITIONAL BENEFITS:** Magnesium relaxes muscles, so it is useful for sports injuries, chronic fatigue and fibromyalgia. It also seems to ease PMS and menstrual cramps, and may increase bone density in postmenopausal women, helping to stem the onset of osteoporosis. In addition, magnesium expands airways, which aids in the treatment of asthma and bronchitis. Studies are inconclusive about magnesium's role in preventing or treating migraines, but one study says it may improve the effect of sumatriptan, a prescription drug used for migraines.

How much you need

The recommended daily amount for magnesium is 300 mg for men and 270 mg for women. Higher doses are required for teenage girls (300 mg) and for disease prevention or treatment.

⊟ **IF YOU GET TOO LITTLE:** Even moderate deficiencies can increase the risk of heart disease and diabetes. Severe deficiencies can result in irregular heartbeat, fatigue, muscle spasms, irritability, nervousness and confusion.

⊞ **IF YOU GET TOO MUCH:** Magnesium may cause diarrhoea and nausea. More serious side effects – including muscle weakness, lethargy, confusion and difficulty in breathing – can develop if the body is unable to process high doses properly. Large amounts lower blood pressure. and may therefore cause dizziness. But overdoses of magnesium are rare because absorption decreases as intake increases, and because the kidneys are usually efficient at eliminating excess amounts.

How to take it

▨ **DOSAGE:** *For heart disease prevention*: Take 300 mg a day. *For arrythmias, asthma and recovery from heart failure*: Use 300 mg a day. *For chronic fatigue*: Take 150 mg of magnesium, preferably as magnesium citrate, twice a day. *For diabetes and high blood pressure*: Take 300 mg a day.

◉ **GUIDELINES FOR USE:** Magnesium is best absorbed when taken with each meal. If supplements cause diarrhoea, lower the dose or try magnesium glucomate, which has a gentler effect on the digestive tract.

Other sources

Good food sources of magnesium are whole grains, nuts, legumes, dark green leafy vegetables and shellfish.

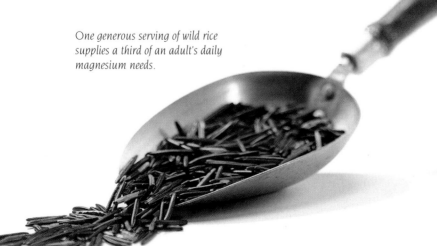

One generous serving of wild rice supplies a third of an adult's daily magnesium needs.

Milk thistle

Silybum marianum

The medicinal use of milk thistle can be traced back to ancient Greece and Rome. Today researchers around the world have completed more than 300 scientific studies that attest to the benefits of this herb, particularly in the treatment of liver ailments.

Common uses

- Protects liver from toxins, including drugs, poisons and chemicals.
- Treats liver disorders such as cirrhosis and hepatitis.
- Reduces liver damage from excessive alcohol.
- Aids in the treatment and prevention of gallstones.
- Helps to clear psoriasis.

Forms

- Capsule
- Softgel
- Tablet
- Tincture

CAUTION!

- Any liver disease requires careful evaluation and treatment by a doctor.

REMINDER: If you have a medical condition, consult your doctor before taking supplements.

What it is

Known by its botanical name, *Silybum marianum*, as well as by its main active ingredient, silymarin, milk thistle is a member of the sunflower family, with purple flowers and milky white leaf veins. The herb blooms from June to August, and the shiny black seeds used for medicinal purposes are collected at the end of summer.

What it does

Milk thistle is one of the most extensively studied and documented herbs in use today. Scientific research continues to validate its healing powers, particularly for the treatment of liver-related disorders. Most of its effectiveness stems from a complex of three liver-protecting compounds, collectively known as silymarin, which constitutes 4% to 6% of the ripe seeds.

MAJOR BENEFITS: Among the benefits of milk thistle is its ability to fortify the liver, one of the body's most important organs. The liver processes nutrients, including fats and other foods. In addition it neutralises, or detoxifies, many drugs, chemical pollutants and alcohol. Milk thistle helps to enhance and strengthen the liver by preventing the depletion of glutathione, an amino acid-like compound that is essential to the detoxifying process. Moreover, studies have shown that it can increase glutathione concentration by up to 35%. Milk thistle is an effective gatekeeper, limiting the number of toxins which the liver processes at any given time. The herb is also a powerful antioxidant. Even more potent than vitamins C and E, it helps to prevent damage

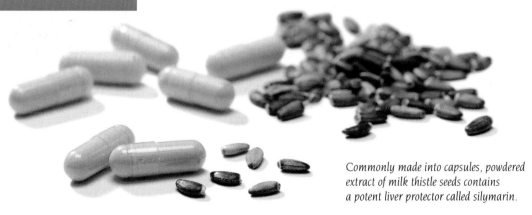

Commonly made into capsules, powdered extract of milk thistle seeds contains a potent liver protector called silymarin.

from highly reactive free-radical molecules. It promotes the regeneration of healthy new liver cells which replace old and damaged ones. Milk thistle eases a range of serious liver ailments, including viral infections (hepatitis) and scarring of the liver (cirrhosis). The herb is so potent that it is sometimes given in an injectable form in hospitable resuscitation rooms to combat the life-threatening, liver-obliterating effects of poisonous mushrooms. In addition, because excessive alcohol depletes glutathione, milk thistle can aid in protecting the livers of alcoholics or those recovering from alcohol abuse.

⊛ **ADDITIONAL BENEFITS:** In cancer patients, milk thistle limits the potential for drug-induced damage to the liver after chemotherapy, and it speeds recovery by hastening the removal of toxic substances that can accumulate in the body. The herb also reduces the inflammation and may slow the skin-cell proliferation associated with psoriasis. It may be useful for endometriosis (the most common cause of infertility in women) because it helps the liver to process the hormone oestrogen, which at high levels can make pain and other symptoms worse. Finally, milk thistle can be beneficial in preventing or treating gallstones by improving the flow of bile, the cholesterol-laden digestive juice that travels from the liver through the gall bladder and into the intestine, where it helps to digest fats.

How to take it

⃠ **DOSAGE:** The recommended dose for milk thistle is up to 200 mg of standardised extract (containing 70% to 80% silymarin) three times a day; lower doses are often very effective. It is often combined with other herbs and nutrients, such as dandelion, choline, methionine and inositol. This combination may be labelled 'liver complex' or 'lipotropic factors' ('lipotropic' refers to the formula's fat-metabolising properties; it prevents the build-up of fatty substances in the liver). For proper dosage follow the instructions on the packet.

◉ **GUIDELINES FOR USE:** Milk thistle extract seems most effective when taken between meals. However, if you want to take the herb itself, a tablespoon of ground milk thistle can be sprinkled over breakfast cereal, once daily. Milk thistle's benefits may be noticeable within a week or two, though long-term treatment is often needed for chronic conditions. The herb appears to be safe, even for pregnant and breastfeeding women. No interactions with other medications have been noted.

Possible side effects

Virtually no side effects have been attributed to the use of milk thistle, which is considered one of the safest herbs on the market. However, in some people it may have a slight laxative effect for a day or two.

RECENT FINDINGS

Milk thistle may be a weapon in the fight against skin cancer. Researchers at Case Western Reserve University in Cleveland, Ohio, found that when the active ingredient, silymarin, was applied to the skin of mice, 75% fewer skin tumours resulted after the mice were exposed to ultra-violet radiation. More studies are needed to see if it has a similar effect in humans.

DID YOU KNOW?

The components of milk thistle are not very soluble in water, so teas made from the seeds usually contain few of the herb's liver-protecting ingredients.

Nettle

Urtica dioica

The healing powers of this herb were recognised by the ancient Greeks. One of its early uses was to remove venom from snakebites. Modern research shows that nettle leaf has a valuable role to play in treating eczema and hay fever, as well as in easing the pain and inflammation of gout.

Common uses

- *Helps to reduce inflammation caused by eczema and skin rashes, and to relieve inflamed joints.*
- *Helps the body to eliminate excess fluid, and alleviates urinary tract infections.*
- *Relieves allergy symptoms, particularly hay fever.*
- *May ease prostate symptoms.*

Forms

- Capsule
- Dried herb/tea
- Liquid
- Tincture

CAUTION!

REMINDER: If you have a medical condition, consult your doctor before taking supplements.

What it is

Strange as it may seem, the original interest in using nettle for medicinal purposes was probably inspired by the plant's ability to irritate exposed skin. Nettle leaves are covered with tiny hairs – hollow needles actually – that sting and burn upon contact. This effect was believed to be beneficial for joint pain (stinging oneself with nettle is an old folk remedy for arthritis), and for centuries nettle leaf poultices were applied to draw toxins from the skin.

Nettle leaves are also considered a nutritious food, and taste like spinach. They are particularly high in iron and other minerals and are rich in carotenoids and vitamin C. (Select young shoots, which have no stingers.) Found in parts of Europe, the USA and Canada, the plant often grows up to 1½ metres high.

What it does

Nettle leaf has valuable cleansing, detoxifying and diuretic properties, possibly owing to its high content of flavonoids and potassium. It is therefore helpful for alleviating many skin conditions, including childhood eczema, and the arthritic problems of later life. Stinging yourself with nettle leaves probably won't help your joint pain, but nettle tea applied as a compress or nettle supplements taken orally may relieve inflamed joints, especially in people with gout.

MAJOR BENEFITS: As a diuretic, nettle helps the body rid itself of excess fluid, and it may be useful as an auxiliary treatment for many disorders. People suffering from urinary tract infections, for example,

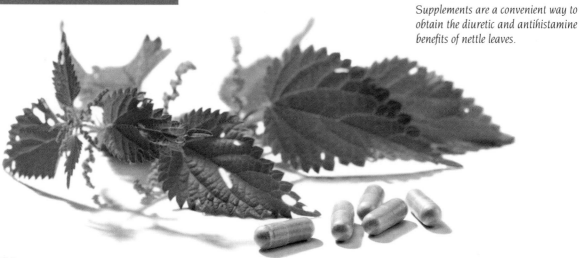

Supplements are a convenient way to obtain the diuretic and antihistamine benefits of nettle leaves.

may find that it promotes urination, which flushes infection-causing bacteria out of the body. Women who become bloated just before their periods may experience some relief after taking nettle supplements.

One of the tried-and-tested benefits of nettle leaf is its ability to control hay fever symptoms. Nasal congestion and watery eyes result when the body produces an inflammatory compound called histamine in response to pollen and other allergens. Nettle is a good source of quercetin, a flavonoid that has been shown to inhibit the release of histamine. In one study of allergy sufferers, more than half of the participants rated nettle moderately to highly effective in reducing allergy symptoms when compared with a placebo.

❉ **ADDITIONAL BENEFITS:** Nettle leaf, taken internally, has an astringent action, and so helps to stop bleeding; it is used to treat nosebleeds and heavy menstrual bleeding.

Nettle root – rather than leaf – may be useful for men with enlarged prostate glands, when this is not caused by cancer. This condition, called benign prostatic hyperplasia (BPH), occurs when the prostate enlarges and narrows the urethra (the tube that transports urine out of the bladder), making urination difficult; diagnosis should be established by a doctor. Nettle root may aid in slowing prostate growth.

How to take it

🖉 **DOSAGE:** *For fluid retention, allergies, eczema, excessive bleeding and gout:* Drink one cup of nettle tea three times a day; use 1 teaspoon of the dried herb per 250 ml of very hot water. Alternatively, take 250 mg extract three times a day, or one teaspoon of tincture three times a day. You can also apply a compress of nettle tea to painful joints. *For slowing prostate growth in* BPH: Take 250 mg nettle root (not leaf) extract twice a day, in combination with 160 mg of saw palmetto extract.

◉ **GUIDELINES FOR USE:** Take nettle leaf (leaves, extract or tincture) with food to minimise the risk of stomach upset. If you want to try the fresh leaves as a vegetable, keep in mind that the young shoots can be eaten raw, but older leaves (with mature, stinging hairs) must be cooked to deactivate the stingers.

Possible side effects

Generally, nettle is considered safe, with only a minimal risk of causing an allergic reaction. There have been some reports, however, that it may irritate the stomach, causing indigestion and diarrhoea.

RECENT FINDINGS

In a preliminary study, nettle helped arthritis patients to cut down on painkillers and reduced the side effects of the drugs. No difference was found in pain, stiffness or the level of physical impairment between patients on 200 mg of the anti-inflammatory drug diclofenac (the brand name is Voltaren) and those taking 50 mg of the drug who also ate 50 grams of nettle leaves each day. In previous studies, lowering the diclofenac dose by just 25% lessened the drug's effectiveness in controlling the symptoms of arthritis.

Niacin

Severe deficiency of this B vitamin, also called nicotinamide and vitamin B_3, results in the debilitating disease pellagra, still found in some developing countries. In the western world niacin is used in the prevention and treatment of depression, arthritis and a host of other ailments.

Common uses

- *May improve circulation.*
- *May ease symptoms of arthritis.*
- *May relieve depression.*
- *May prevent progression of type II diabetes.*

Forms

- Capsule
- Tablet

What it is

The chemical structure of niacin is similar to that of the amino acid tryptophan – found in eggs, meat and poultry – and the body is able to obtain about half its niacin requirements by converting it from the chemical ingredients of tryptophan. The remainder has to come directly from the diet; many protein-rich foods are good sources. In addition, niacin can be obtained from dietary supplements and also from the many cereal products that have been fortified with this and other vitamins.

What it does

Niacin is needed to release energy from carbohydrate foods. It is also involved in controlling blood sugar, keeping skin healthy and maintaining the proper functioning of the nervous and digestive systems. The form of niacin usually sold in the UK is nicotinamide.

PREVENTION: In the 1940s and 1950s there were reports of very good clinical results when high doses of nicotinamide were used to treat people with rheumatoid arthritis and osteoarthritis. Within a few months there were improvements in joint function, range of motion, muscle strength and endurance. These findings have been confirmed by more recent studies. It appears that nicotinamide has an anti-inflammatory effect on these conditions and may help to heal damaged cartilage.

ADDITIONAL BENEFITS: Niacin helps to foster healthy brain and nerve cells, and there is some evidence to indicate that nicotinamide can ease depression, anxiety and insomnia. High doses of nicotinamide may reverse the development of type I diabetes – the form that typically appears before the age of 30 – if it is given early enough. However, this therapy should be tried only under medical supervision.

How much you need

The recommended daily amount of niacin intake is 13 mg for women and 17 mg for men. Far higher doses are required for the effective treatment of various disorders, when niacin is being used as a medication rather than a nutrient.

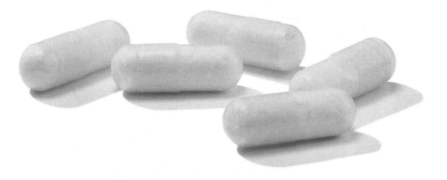

⊖ **IF YOU GET TOO LITTLE:** A slight niacin deficiency results in patches of irritated skin, appetite loss, indigestion and weakness. Severe deficiencies – which are practically nonexistent in industrialised countries – result in pellagra, a debilitating disease. Symptoms include a rash in areas exposed to sunlight, vomiting, a bright red tongue, fatigue and memory loss.

⊕ **IF YOU GET TOO MUCH:** Niacin in the form of nicotinamide presents no danger when taken at the levels normally recommended for dietary supplementation. The upper safe limit is 500 mg daily, When high intakes are regularly prescribed by a doctor, it is necessary for a check to be kept on liver function because too much niacin over a long period of time can damage this organ.

How to take it

☑ **DOSAGE:** *For anxiety and depression:* Take 50 mg of niacin a day; this dose can usually be found as part of a B-complex vitamin. *For insomnia:* Take 500 mg nicotinamide one hour before bedtime. *For arthritis:* Take 500 mg nicotinamide three times a day, but ensure that this treatment is administered only under the supervision of a doctor.

◉ **GUIDELINES FOR USE:** It is best to take niacin with meals to decrease the likelihood of stomach upset, especially at high doses. Do not take therapeutic doses of any form of niacin if you take cholesterol-lowering prescription drugs.

Other sources

Niacin is found in foods that are high in protein, such as chicken, beef, fish and nuts. Breads, cereals and some pasta are also enriched with niacin. Although they are low in niacin, eggs, milk and other dairy products are good alternative sources of the vitamin because they are high in tryptophan.

Many people obtain their daily requirement of niacin from fortified breakfast cereals.

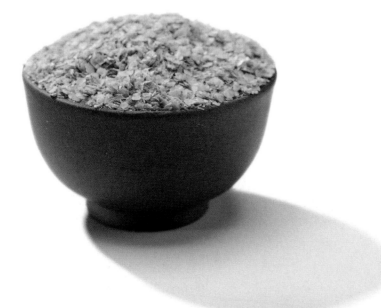

Pau d'arco

Tabebuia impetiginosa

Rumoured to have been prescribed by the Incas to treat serious ailments, the herb pau d'arco has been investigated as a remedy for infectious diseases and cancer. Although its anticancer properties have not yet been confirmed, it may indeed combat a variety of infections.

Common uses

- *Treats thrush.*
- *Helps to get rid of warts.*
- *Reduces inflammation of the airways in bronchitis.*
- *May be useful in treating such immune-related disorders as asthma, eczema, psoriasis and bacterial and viral infections.*

Forms

- Capsule
- Dried herb/tea
- Powder
- Softgel
- Tablet
- Tincture

CAUTION!

- **Pregnant or breastfeeding women should avoid pau d'arco.**
- **Pau d'arco may duplicate the effect of anticoagulant drugs.**

REMINDER: If you have a medical condition, consult your doctor before taking supplements.

What it is

Pau d'arco is obtained from the inner bark of a tree – *Tabebuia impetiginosa* – indigenous to the rain forests of South America. Native tribes have taken advantage of its healing powers for centuries. Pau d'arco is also known as *lapacho*, taheebo or *ipe roxo*. In the UK, however, it is always sold as pau d'arco.

The therapeutic ingredients in pau d'arco include a host of potent plant chemicals called naphthoquinones. Of these, lapachol has been the most intensely studied.

What it does

Lapachol and other compounds in pau d'arco help to destroy the microorganisms that cause diseases and infections, from malaria and flu to thrush. Most people, however, are interested in the potential cancer-fighting properties of the herb.

MAJOR BENEFITS: Pau d'arco appears to combat bacteria, viruses and fungi, reduce inflammation and support the immune system. One of its best-documented uses is for the treatment of thrush; herbalists often recommend a pau d'arco tea douche to restore the normal environment of the vagina. In capsule, tablet, tincture or tea form pau d'arco may be effective in strengthening immunity in cases of chronic fatigue syndrome, chronic bronchitis, or HIV and AIDS. The herb's anti-inflammatory properties likewise may help to treat acute bronchitis, which involves inflammation of the respiratory passages, as well as muscle pain. A directly applied tincture of pau d'arco can eradicate warts.

ADDITIONAL BENEFITS: Pau d'arco's anticancer activity is subject to continuing debate. Because of the herb's traditional reputation as a cancer fighter the US National Cancer Institute (NCI) investigated it, identifying lapachol as its most active ingredient. In animal studies pau

Pau d'arco can be taken as a supplement or brewed as a tea.

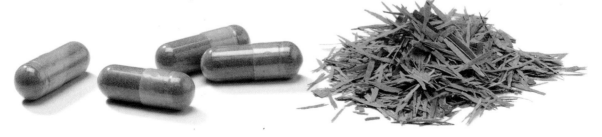

d'arco showed promise in shrinking tumours, and so in the 1970s the NCI began human trials using high doses of lapachol. Again there was some evidence that lapachol was active in destroying cancer cells, but participants taking a therapeutic dose suffered serious side effects, including nausea, vomiting and blood-clotting problems. As a result, research into lapachol and its source, pau d'arco, was abandoned.

Critics of this investigation believe that using therapeutic doses of pau d'arco – and not simply the isolated compound lapachol – would have produced similar benefits without the potentially dangerous blood-thinning effects. It's likely that lapachol interferes with the action of vitamin K, needed for the blood to clot properly. Some researchers suggest that other compounds in pau d'arco supply some vitamin K, so that use of the whole herb would not interfere with blood clotting. Others think that combining lapachol with vitamin K supplements might make it possible for people to take doses of lapachol high enough to permit its potential anti-tumour action to be studied further without provoking a reaction. Despite the controversy many practitioners rely on the historical evidence of pau d'arco's anticancer action and often recommend it as a complement to conventional cancer treatment.

How to take it

DOSAGE: When pau d'arco is used in capsule or tablet form the typical dosage is 250 mg of the powered herb twice a day. This dose of pau d'arco is often recommended for chronic fatigue syndrome, or HIV and AIDS, in alternation with other immune-boosting herbs such as echinacea or goldenseal. Pau d'arco is also commonly taken as a tea in dried herb form. To make it, steep 2 or 3 teaspoons of pau d'arco in 500 ml of very hot water; drink the tea over the course of a day.

GUIDELINES FOR USE: Herbalists recommend using whole-bark products (not only those that contain just lapachol) because they suspect that the herb's healing properties come from the full range of plant chemicals in the bark. *For vaginal yeast infections*: Let pau d'arco tea cool to lukewarm before using it as a douche. *For warts*: Apply a tincture-soaked compress to the affected area at bedtime and leave it on all night. Repeat until the wart disappears. Seek advice from your doctor if you suffer from genital warts.

Possible side effects

Whole-bark products are generally safe; they do not produce the side effects of high doses of lapachol. If pau d'arco tea or supplements cause stomach upset, take them with food.

Peppermint

Mentha piperita

For centuries this powerfully aromatic herb has provided relief for indigestion, colds and headaches. Today medicinal peppermint is most highly prized for its ability to soothe the digestive tract, easing indigestion, irritable bowel syndrome and other abdominal complaints.

Common uses

- *Relieves nausea and indigestion.*
- *Eases symptoms of diverticulitis and irritable bowel syndrome.*
- *Helps to dissolve gallstones.*
- *Sweetens the breath.*
- *Soothes muscle aches.*
- *Eases coughs and congestion caused by allergies or colds.*

Forms

- Capsule
- Dried or fresh herb/tea
- Oil
- Ointment/cream
- Tincture

CAUTION!

- Peppermint oil relaxes gastrointestinal muscles, so it may aggravate the symptoms of a hiatus hernia.

- Peppermint oil should not be applied to the nostrils or chests of infants and children under the age of five because it can cause a choking sensation.

REMINDER: If you have a medical condition, consult your doctor before taking supplements.

What it is

Peppermint is cultivated worldwide for use as a flavouring and a herbal medicine. A natural hybrid of spearmint and water mint, peppermint has square stems, pointed dark green or purple oval leaves and lilac-coloured flowers. For medicinal purposes, the leaves and stems of the plant are harvested just before the flowers bloom in summer. The major active ingredient of peppermint is its volatile oil, which is made up of more than 40 different compounds. The oil's therapeutic effect comes mainly from menthol (35% to 55% of the oil), menthone (15% to 30%) and menthyl acetate (3% to 10%). Medicinal peppermint oil is made by steam-distilling the parts of the plant that grow above the ground.

What it does

Particularly effective in treating digestive disorders, peppermint relieves cramps and relaxes intestinal muscles. It freshens the breath and may clear up nasal congestion as well.

✤ **MAJOR BENEFITS:** Peppermint oil relaxes the muscles of the digestive tract, helping to relieve intestinal cramping and gas. Its antispasmodic effect also makes it useful for alleviating the symptoms of irritable bowel syndrome, a common disorder characterised by abdominal pain, alternating bouts of diarrhoea and constipation, and indigestion. The menthol in peppermint aids digestion because it stimulates the flow of natural digestive juices and bile. This action explains why peppermint oil

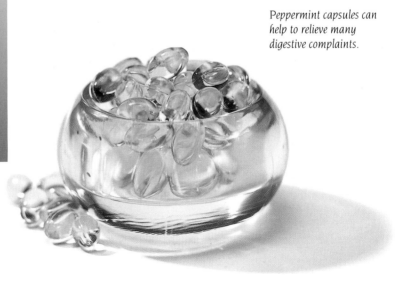

Peppermint capsules can help to relieve many digestive complaints.

is commonly included in over-the-counter antacids. Several studies show that the menthol in peppermint oil also assists in dissolving gallstones, providing a possible alternative to surgery. Consult your doctor before trying the oil for this purpose. You can also put the oil directly on your tongue; it provides a minty antidote to bad breath.

As a tea or an oil, peppermint serves as a mild anaesthetic to the stomach's mucous lining, which helps to reduce nausea and motion sickness. The tea may ease symptoms of diverticulitis as well, including flatulence and bloating.

❋ **ADDITIONAL BENEFITS:** When rubbed on the skin, peppermint oil relieves pain by stimulating the nerves that perceive cold while muting those that sense pain, which makes it a good remedy for aching muscles.

Results of studies into peppermint's traditional use in the treatment of colds and coughs are contradictory. Some tests show that the plant has no effect, but Commission E, a German health board recognised as an authority on the scientific investigation of herbs, found that it was an effective decongestant that reduced inflammation of the nasal passageways. Many people with colds report that inhaling peppermint's menthol enables them to breathe more easily. Peppermint tea also may offer relief from the bronchial constriction of asthma.

How to take it

⬚ **DOSAGE:** *For the treatment of irritable bowel syndrome, nausea and gallstones*: Do not ingest peppermint oil itself; enteric-coated capsules release peppermint oil where it's most needed – in the small and large intestine rather than in the stomach. Take one or two capsules (containing 0.2 ml of oil per capsule) two or three times a day, between meals. *To freshen the breath*: Place a few drops of peppermint oil on the tongue. *To relieve flatulence and calm the stomach*: Make a tea by steeping 1 or 2 teaspoons of dried peppermint leaves in 250 ml of very hot water for between 5 and 10 minutes; be sure to cover the cup to prevent the volatile oil from escaping. *For congestion*: Drink up to four cups of peppermint tea a day. *For pain relief*: Add a few drops of peppermint oil to 45 ml (3 tablespoons) of a neutral oil. Apply to the affected areas up to four times daily.

◉ **GUIDELINES FOR USE:** Take enteric-coated capsules between meals. If you prefer peppermint tea, drink a cup three or four times a day, after or between meals. Apply peppermint oil or ointments containing menthol no more than three or four times daily. To take peppermint tincture, put 10 to 20 drops in a glass of water. Peppermint oil should not be used if you are taking homoeopathic treatment, and avoid it during pregnancy.

Possible side effects

Peppermint in the recommended doses generally has no side effects, even when taken for long periods. There have been rare instances of skin rashes and indigestion caused by enteric-coated peppermint oil capsules. Topical peppermint oil can produce allergic skin rashes, especially if heat is being applied as well. If side effects occur, stop using the herb.

Phosphorus

The main function of phosphorus is to interact with calcium to build and maintain strong bones and teeth, but the mineral also plays an essential role in the process of supplying energy to every cell in the body. Fortunately, the likelihood of deficiency is very small.

Common uses

- *Builds strong bones and maintains skeletal integrity.*
- *Helps to form tooth enamel and strengthens teeth.*

Forms

- Capsule
- Liquid
- Powder
- Tablet

CAUTION!

■ The greatest risk associated with phosphorus may be getting too much, which can lead to a calcium deficiency. Never take phosphorus supplements without discussing it with your doctor first.

■ In a rare instance of a phosphorus deficiency – such as from kidney or digestive disease or severe burns – phosphorus supplementation must be medically supervised.

REMINDER: If you have a medical condition, consult your doctor before taking supplements.

What it is

Phosphorus is the second most abundant mineral in the body after calcium, and up to 650 grams of it are found in the average person. Although 85% of this mineral is concentrated in the bones and teeth, the rest is distributed in the blood and in various organs, including the heart, kidneys, brain and muscles. Phosphorus interacts with a variety of other nutrients, but its most constant companion is calcium. In the bones the ratio of calcium to phosphorus is around 2:1. In other tissues, however, the ratio of phosphorus to calcium is much higher.

What it does

There is hardly a biological or cellular process that does not, directly or indirectly, involve phosphorus. In some instances the mineral works to protect cells, strengthening the membranes that surround them; in other cases it acts as a kind of biological escort, assisting a variety of nutrients, hormones and chemicals in doing their jobs. There is also evidence that phosphorus helps to activate the B vitamins and enables them to provide all their benefits.

✪ **MAJOR BENEFITS:** One of phosphorus's most important functions is to team up with calcium to build bones and aid in maintaining a healthy, strong skeleton. The phosphorus-calcium partnership is also crucial for strengthening the teeth and keeping them strong. In addition phosphorus joins with fats in the blood to make compounds called phospholipids which, in turn, play structural and metabolic roles in cell membranes throughout the body. Furthermore, without phosphorus the body could not convert the proteins, carbohydrates and fats from food into energy. The mineral is needed to create the molecule known as adenosine triphosphate, or ATP, which acts like a tiny battery charger, supplying vital energy to every cell in the body.

✪ **ADDITIONAL BENEFITS:** Phosphorus serves as a cell-to-cell messenger. In this capacity it contributes to the coordination of such body processes as muscle contraction, the transmission of nerve impulses from the brain

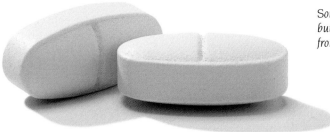

Some multivitamin pills contain phosphorus, but most people get enough of this mineral from their daily diet.

to the body and the secretion of hormones. An adequate phosphorus supply may therefore enhance physical performance and be effective in fighting fatigue. The mineral is necessary for maintaining the pH (the acid-base balance) of the blood and for manufacturing DNA and RNA, the basic components of our genetic makeup.

How much you need

Phosphorus is found in so many foods that the need for supplements is virtually nonexistent. The recommended target for phosphorus in men and women is the same, 550 mg daily. In the past many nutritionists recommended that phosphorus and calcium be taken in a 1:1 ratio, but most recently practitioners have advised that this ratio has little practical benefit. Most people today consume more phosphorus than calcium in their diets.

⊟ **IF YOU GET TOO LITTLE:** Although rare, a deficiency of phosphorus can lead to fragile bones and teeth, fatigue, weakness, a loss of appetite, joint pain and stiffness, and an increased susceptibility to infection. A mild deficiency may produce a modest decrease in energy.

⊞ **IF YOU GET TOO MUCH:** There are no immediate adverse effects from getting too much phosphorus. In the long term, excessive intake of phosphorus may inhibit calcium absorption, though it is uncertain whether this can result in a calcium deficiency that threatens bone health.

How to take it

▨ **DOSAGE:** Most people get all the phosphorus they require in their everyday diets. In addition a small amount of phosphorus may be included in daily multivitamin and mineral supplements. If you have a medical condition that depletes this mineral, such as a bowel ailment or failing kidneys, your doctor will prescribe an appropriate dose.

◉ **GUIDELINES FOR USE:** Never take individual phosphorus supplements except on medical advice.

Other sources

High-protein foods, such as meat, fish, poultry and dairy products, contain a lot of phosphorus. It is also used as an additive in many processed foods. Soft drinks, particularly colas, often have large amounts. Phosphorus is present in grain products as well, although wholegrain breads and cereals may include ingredients that partially reduce its absorption.

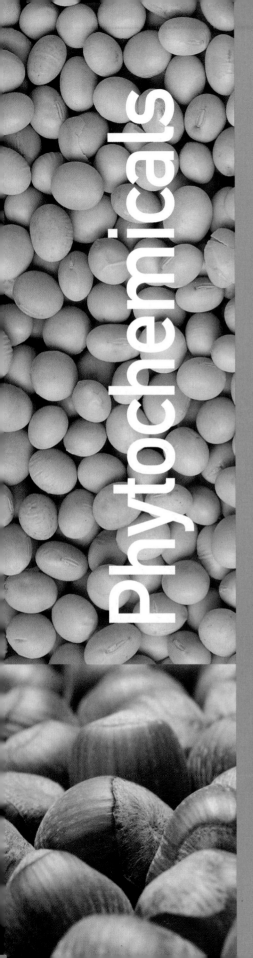

Phytochemicals

Phytochemicals are compounds naturally present in plants. They are neither vitamins, trace minerals nor dietary fibre, but are nevertheless biologically active in the human body. In recent years they have generated particular interest as a result of their potential benefits to health. While most research has focused on fruit and vegetables as sources of phytochemicals, similar substances are found in culinary and medicinal herbs.

Phytochemicals have been shown to have complementary and overlapping effects on the human body. As well as a host of antioxidant, antibacterial and antiviral actions, these include:

■ Stimulating liver enzymes that deal with and help to get rid of toxins.
■ Stimulating the functioning of the immune system.
■ Reducing the danger of blood clots.
■ Regulating cholesterol levels and hormone metabolism.
■ Reducing blood pressure.

ANTIOXIDANT EFFECTS

Most phytochemicals have powerful antioxidant properties, good examples being flavonoids and carotenoids. This means they are able to neutralise free radicals, the unstable molecules that can cause cell damage.

The antioxidant action of phytochemicals is believed to reduce the risk of heart disease and to limit the development of inflammation in tissues that are being damaged by free radicals. For example, quercetin (found in onions and apples) has an anti-inflammatory action that may help to alleviate allergic respiratory reactions such as hay fever and asthma, skin conditions such as eczema, and inflammatory disorders of the joints and muscles.

FLAVONOIDS

Flavonoids (or bioflavonoids) are a large group of phyto-chemicals, examples of which are found in all plants. Most are colourless, but some are responsible for the bright colours of many fruits and vegetables. The human diet usually includes at least 1 gram per day of flavonoids, and tea and wines (especially red) contain large quantities.

More than 4000 flavonoids have been identified so far, and many of them have been intensively investigated by laboratory and animal studies. Except for one major flavonoid – quercetin – few have been the subject of human studies.

Rutin and hesperidin – found in buckwheat and citrus fruit, respectively – are among the most potent antioxidant flavonoids. Chemical subgroups of flavonoids include OPCs (oligomeric proanthocyanidins, which are abundant in grape seed extract), isoflavones (in soya) and anthocyanosides (the red pigment in, for example, red wines and blackberries).

Other pigments found in plants are the carotenoids, which give red, orange and yellow colours. Unlike the flavonoid pigments they are fat soluble, so the yellow colour of butter is due to beta-carotene from grass eaten by cows.

CABBAGES AND ONIONS

There are two important groups of sulphur-containing phytochemicals. Glucosinolates, believed to provide protection against cancer, are found in all members of the cabbage family, including broccoli, cauliflower and Brussels sprouts.

The onion family contains several closely related sulphur compounds with health benefits – garlic is an especially rich source.

HERBS THAT CONTAIN PHYTOCHEMICALS

As well as being rich sources of flavonoids, most herbs – and particularly herbal medicines – contain phytochemicals that are either protective or have curative properties. For example, liquorice and ginseng (and also soya) contain saponins that are chemically similar to the body's steroids.

Other herbs contain active constituents that are unique to the plant, and are often named accordingly: ginkgolides from ginkgo, echinoside from echinacea, valerenic acid from valerian, and so on.

THE POWER OF PHYTOESTROGENS

The principal phytoestrogens in the human diet are the isoflavones and a group of compounds called lignans, found in rye bran, flaxseed, sesame seeds and nuts.

Most research has been undertaken into isoflavones, which occur almost exclusively in legumes – soya beans are the most important dietary source. The main isoflavones found in soya proteins and soya foods are daidzein, genistein and glycitein.

Although not chemically related, phytoestrogens have some similarities to the female sex hormone oestrodiol, produced by women's bodies, which allows them to bind to oestrogen 'receptors' in cells.

Phytoestrogens will have no effect on the level of blood oestrogen, but by binding to these receptors they have an oestrogenic (oestrogen-like) effect when the hormone is lacking and an anti-oestrogenic effect when it is in excess.

Oestrogen also circulates in men's blood and high levels are associated with increased risk of cancer of the prostate gland. Soya phytoestrogens are believed to have a protective effect against prostate cancer.

The level of oestrogen in a woman's body falls after the menopause. At this time phytoestrogens are thought to provide a substitute for the body's own oestrogen, and may help to relieve symptoms such as hot flushes and dry skin. Phytoestrogens may also help to reduce the loss of bone mineral density that normally occurs after the menopause and is associated with osteoporosis.

THE ASIAN DIET

In Asian countries such as Japan, where the diet is rich in soya foods, menopausal symptoms such as hot flushes are reported much less than in Western countries. For example, in Europe 70-80% of menopausal women experience hot flushes, compared with 57% in Malaysia and 18% in China. One of the

A THERAPEUTIC DOSE OF ISOFLAVONES

Not enough is known about isoflavones to be able to recommend a daily amount, but consumption of isoflavones in Asia is between 25 and 200 mg a day. An intake of 50 to 120 mg isoflavones a day may be needed for therapeutic effects. On average this can be provided by one or two portions of soya products a day, but the isoflavone content is very variable.

The following foods yield approximately 50 mg isoflavones:
- 100 grams firm tofu or 200 grams soft tofu
- 100 grams miso
- 250 ml soya milk or soya yoghurt
- 50 grams soya flour, cooked soya beans or textured vegetable protein (TVP)

Most soya proteins used by the food industry contain 10-300 mg isoflavones per 100 grams. Soy sauce, soya bean oil and lecithin contain virtually no isoflavones.

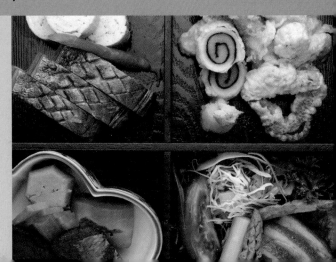

THE MAIN GROUPS OF PHYTOCHEMICALS: WHERE THEY COME FROM AND WHAT THEY DO

PHYTOCHEMICAL GROUPS	EXAMPLES OF COMPOUNDS	MAIN FOOD SOURCES	ACTION
Flavonoids	Kaempferol, quercetin Hesperitin, naringenin, rutin, tangeritin	Artichoke, apples, lettuce, onions, peppers, tea, tomatoes, wine; citrus fruits: grapefruit, oranges, tangerines	Antioxidants; enzyme regulators May prevent cancer and cardiovascular disease; may regulate immunity
Glucosinolates/ Isothiocyanates	Allylisothiocyanates, glucobrassicin, indoles	Cabbage family (broccoli, Brussels sprouts, cauliflower), mustard, watercress	Liver enzyme inducers; may prevent cancer
Hydroxycinnamic acids	Caffeic, chlorogenic and ferulic acids, curcumin	Apples, coffee, curry powder, mustard, pears	Antioxidants; may prevent cancer
Isoflavones	Daidzein, genistein	Soya bean products (soya flour, soya milk, soya protein)	Lower serum lipids; anti-oestrogenic; may prevent breast and prostate cancers
Lignans	Matairesinoll, secoisolaciresinol	Berries, flaxseed, nuts, rye bran	Antioxidant and antioestrogenic effects; may prevent colon and prostate cancers
Monoterpenes	D-carvone, D-limonene, perrillyl alcohol	Cherries, citrus fruits, herbs (dill, mint, caraway)	Liver enzyme inducers; anti-tumour agents (especially in respect of breast, prostate and pancreas), antimicrobial
Organosulphides	Allyl methyl sulphide, diallyl sulphide	Cabbage, garlic, leeks, onions, etc	Reduce blood clotting; lowers blood lipids; liver enzyme inducers; may prevent cancer
Phenols	Ellagic acid, gallic acid, hydroquinone, ρ-cresol	Widespread, including black tea, cocoa beans, green tea, raspberries, strawberries	Antioxidants; anti-inflammatory agents
Phytosterols	B-sitosterol, campesterol, stigmasterol	Vegetable oils (corn, rapeseed, soya bean, sunflower); specialist margarines (such as Benecol) contain ten times as much	Lower total cholesterol and LDL ('bad') cholesterol
Tannins	Theaflavins, thearubigens	Black tea, red wine, roasted coffee	Antioxidants; antimicrobial and anti-inflammatory agents

A POWERFUL WEAPON IN THE BATTLE AGAINST CANCER
Death rates for breast cancer in women are around 27.7 per 100,000 women in the UK compared with 6.6 in Japan. Prostate cancer deaths are similarly around four times greater in the UK than in Japan – and these figures are associated with significantly lower intakes of isoflavones.

most striking dietary differences among women in these areas is their intake of dietary soya protein and the phytoestrogens it contains. Japanese women excrete 100-1000 times more oestrogens in their urine than Western women.

In 1998 a study found that menopausal women who added 40 grams of isolated soya protein with naturally occurring isoflavones to their diet experienced a 45% reduction in hot flushes after 12 weeks.

LOWERING THE INCIDENCE OF OSTEOPOROSIS

Osteoporosis is the main underlying cause of most of the 60,000 hip fractures in England and Wales each year. It is incurable, but – along with increased prescribing of hormone replacement therapy (HRT) to help to prevent loss of bone mineral density – there is growing interest in dietary isoflavones as an alternative means of preventing it.

In Asian women the incidence of fractures due to osteoporosis is lower than in the West, despite the fact that Asian women have smaller frames, consume fewer dairy products and have lower calcium intakes.

A recent study of post-menopausal women found a small but significant increase in bone density with a diet containing 90 mg of total isoflavones that came from soya protein. It is thought that the isoflavones in soya may inhibit the breakdown of bone. Synthetic isoflavones with the same structure as those in soya protein are also effective in reducing bone loss.

REDUCING THE LIKELIHOOD OF CANCER

A low consumption of fruit and vegetables is now considered by many scientists to be an important factor in increasing the risk of cancer. A reduced risk of cancer appears to be more strongly linked with the intake of certain foods – fruit, vegetables and legumes – than with intake of the antioxidant vitamins C, E and A, or fibre.

This suggests that other, non-essential substances – such as phytochemicals – play a key role in lowering risk. Drinking tea can help too. Animal studies have shown that green tea

inhibits carcinogenesis (the formation of tumours) in the lung and liver, as well as in the intestine and large bowel.

Death rates for breast cancer and prostate cancer are four times higher in the UK than in Japan, and these differences are linked with significantly lower intakes of isoflavones.

PROTECTION AGAINST HEART DISEASE

The commonest cause of heart disease is atheroscelerosis, or hardening of the arteries by a fatty substance called plaque.

Flavonoids such as OPCs and quercetin can inhibit the process of atherosclerosis and help to strengthen blood vessels; in this way they may protect against heart disease and circulatory disorders. Equally, differences in the consumption of flavonoids may account for about 25% of the variations in heart disease between different countries.

Risk of atherosclerosis may also be reduced by isoflavones. A recent trial found that a daily dose of 62 mg isoflavones, taken as soya protein, reduced LDL 'bad' cholesterol by 10%.

Isoflavones, especially genistein, are also thought to reduce the risk of heart attacks as a result of their anticoagulant properties, which may impede the formation of clots in the blood and so prevent arterial blockages. However, most of the evidence is derived from laboratory and animal studies, and these need to be confirmed with further study on humans.

PHYTOCHEMICALS AS SUPPLEMENTS
Scientific studies have confirmed the centuries-old wisdom that plant foods are highly protective against many different diseases. The health benefits of plants have been mainly attributed to the vitamins and phytochemicals they contain. Phytochemicals from vegetables, fruit and herbs are now readily available as tablets and tinctures. In addition to being used to complement the diet, many of these preparations can be just as effective as their traditional counterparts in restoring an ailing body to good health.

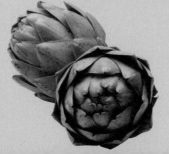

Potassium

You are probably careful not to eat too much salt, especially if you are monitoring your blood pressure levels, but you might also want to increase your consumption of potassium. In some people this mineral may do as much to control blood pressure as reducing sodium intake.

Common uses

- Helps to lower blood pressure.
- May prevent high blood pressure, heart disease and stroke.

Forms

- Liquid
- Powder
- Tablet

CAUTION!

- If you suffer from a kidney disease or are taking medication for high blood pressure or heart disease, do not take potassium supplements without consulting your doctor.

REMINDER: If you have a medical condition, consult your doctor before taking supplements.

What it is

The third most abundant mineral in the body after calcium and phosphorus, potassium is an electrolyte – a substance that takes on a positive or negative charge when dissolved in the watery medium of the bloodstream. Sodium and chloride are electrolytes too, and the body needs a balance of these minerals to perform a host of essential functions. Almost all the potassium in the body is found inside the cells.

What it does

Along with the other electrolytes, potassium is used to conduct nerve impulses, initiate muscle contractions and regulate heartbeat and blood pressure. It controls the amount of fluid inside the cells, and sodium regulates the amount outside, so the two minerals work to balance fluid levels in the body. Potassium also enables the body to convert blood sugar (glucose) – its primary fuel – into a stored form of energy (glycogen) that is held in reserve by the muscles and liver. It is a natural diuretic, so helps to remove toxic metabolites, or toxins, from the body.

🛡 **PREVENTION:** Study after study has shown that people who get plenty of potassium in their diets have lower blood pressure than those who get very little. This effect holds true even when sodium intake remains high (though reducing sodium produces better results). In one study 54 people on medication for high blood pressure were divided into two groups. Half followed their regular diet; the other half added three to six servings of potassium-rich foods a day. After a year 81% of those getting extra potassium were able to reduce their drug dosages significantly, compared with only 29% of the individuals following their regular diets.

✳ **ADDITIONAL BENEFITS:** Through its effects on blood pressure, potassium may also decrease the risk of heart disease and stroke. In one study a group of people with hypertension who ate one serving of a food high in potassium every day reduced their risk of fatal stroke by 40%. A 12-year investigation found that men who got the least amount of

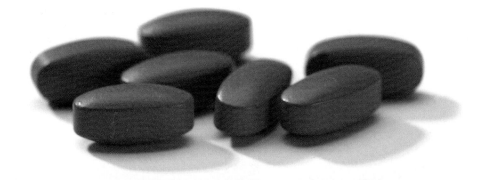

potassium were two and a half times more likely to die from a stroke than men who consumed the most; for women with a low potassium intake, the risk of fatal stroke was nearly five times greater.

How much you need

The recommended target for potassium is 3500 mg a day for both men and women. The mineral is found in a wide variety of foods, fruit and vegetables being particularly rich sources. However, many people do not eat enough of this vital food group, and a third of the UK population has a potassium intake of 2500 mg or less.

⊟ **IF YOU GET TOO LITTLE:** In otherwise healthy people a low intake of potassium is unlikely to produce adverse symptoms. At even lower intakes the first sign of deficiency would be muscle weakness and nausea. A serious deficiency can occur if an individual is taking a potent diuretic (a drug that reduces fluid levels in the body) or is suffering from an extreme case of diarrhoea or vomiting. If potassium is not replaced, such low levels could lead to heart failure.

⊞ **IF YOU GET TOO MUCH:** Potassium toxicity is highly unlikely because most people can safely consume up to 18 grams a day. Toxicity usually occurs only if an individual has a kidney disorder or takes too many potassium supplements. Signs of potassium overload include muscle fatigue and an irregular heartbeat. Even in small doses, potassium supplements may cause stomach irritation and nausea.

How to take it

☑ **DOSAGE:** Most people don't need potassium supplements unless they are taking certain diuretic medications. Try to get sufficient potassium in your daily diet. People who use ACE inhibitors (such as captopril or enalapril) for high blood pressure or angina, and those who have kidney disease, should not take potassium supplements at all.

◉ **GUIDELINES FOR USE:** If you do need to take potassium supplements, take them with food to decrease stomach irritation.

Other sources

Fresh vegetables and fruit – such as potatoes, bananas, oranges and orange juice – are very high in potassium. Meats, poultry, milk and yoghurt are also good sources.

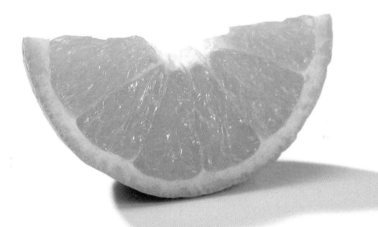

The results of 33 studies show that potassium has a positive impact on blood pressure. People with normal blood pressure who added 2340 mg of potassium a day – from foods, supplements or a combination of both – to their normal diets had an average drop of two points in systolic blood pressure (the upper reading) and one point in diastolic pressure (the lower reading). These small changes reduce by 25% the chance of developing hypertension. The extra potassium offered even greater benefits – a 4.4 point drop in systolic pressure and a 2.5 point drop in diastolic – in people who already had high blood pressure.

DID YOU KNOW?

Sustained exercise depletes the level of potassium in muscles, so athletes must repeatedly replenish their stores of the mineral.

FACTS & TIPS

■ Microwave or steam vegetables whenever you can; boiling them decreases their potassium content. Boiled potatoes lose 50% of their potassium; steamed potatoes lose less than 6%.

■ Potassium supplements should not contain more than 99 mg per tablet (this includes multivitamin and mineral preparations). If you think you need potassium supplements, talk to your doctor about higher-dose pills available on prescription.

Riboflavin

Exciting new research suggests that riboflavin, also known as vitamin B_2, may possess a range of previously unsuspected medicinal powers. It has been credited with counteracting migraines, preventing sight-robbing cataracts, healing skin blemishes – and much more.

Common uses

- Prevents or delays the onset of cataracts.
- Reduces the frequency and severity of migraines.
- Improves skin blemishes caused by rosacea.

Forms

- Capsule
- Tablet

What it is

In 1879 scientists looking through a microscope discovered a fluorescent yellow-green substance in milk, but not until 1933 was it identified as riboflavin. This water-soluble vitamin is part of the B-complex family, which is involved in transforming protein, fats and carbohydrates into fuel for the body. Found naturally in many foods, riboflavin is also added to fortified breads and cereals. It is easily destroyed when exposed to sunlight. Inadequate riboflavin intake often accompanies other B-vitamin deficiencies, which are a common problem in the elderly and alcoholics. Riboflavin is available as a single supplement, in combination with other B vitamins (vitamin B complex), or as part of a multivitamin.

What it does

The body depends on riboflavin for a wide range of functions. It plays a vital role in the production of thyroid hormone, which speeds up metabolism and helps to ensure a steady supply of energy. Riboflavin also aids the body in producing infection-fighting immune cells; it works in conjunction with iron to manufacture red blood cells, which transport oxygen to all the cells in the body. In addition it converts vitamins B_6 and niacin into active forms so that they can do their work.

Riboflavin produces substances that assist antioxidants, such as vitamin E, in protecting cells against damage from the naturally occurring, highly reactive molecules known as free radicals. It is essential for tissue maintenance and repair – the body uses extra amounts to speed the healing of wounds after surgery, burns and other injuries. The vitamin is also necessary to maintain the function of the eyes, and may be important for healthy nerves as well.

◈ **PREVENTION:** By boosting antioxidant activity riboflavin protects many body tissues – particularly the lens of the eye. It may therefore help to prevent the formation of cataracts, the milky opacities in the lenses that impair the vision of so many elderly people. Ophthalmologists urge everyone, especially those with a family history of this eye disorder, to get an adequate, steady supply of riboflavin throughout their lives.

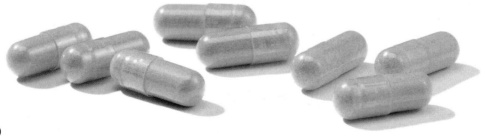

The vitamin has also been shown to be highly effective in reducing the frequency and severity of migraine headaches. Migraine sufferers are believed to have reduced energy reserves in the brain, and riboflavin may prevent attacks by increasing the energy supply to brain cells.

⊕ **ADDITIONAL BENEFITS:** Riboflavin has proved valuable in treating skin disorders including rosacea, which causes facial flushing and skin pustules in many adults. In combination with other B vitamins, including vitamin B_6 and niacin, it may help against a broad range of nerve and other ailments, including numbness and tingling, Alzheimer's disease, epilepsy and multiple sclerosis, as well as anxiety, stress and even fatigue. Some doctors prescribe riboflavin supplementation to treat sickle-cell anaemia because many people with the disease have a riboflavin deficiency.

How much you need

The daily recommended target for riboflavin is 1.3 mg a day for men and 1.1 mg for women. These amounts simply prevent general deficiencies; larger doses are usually prescribed for specific conditions.

⊖ **IF YOU GET TOO LITTLE:** Classic deficiency symptoms include cracking and sores in the corner of the mouth and increased sensitivity to sunlight, with watering, burning and itchy eyes. The skin round the nose, eyebrows and ear lobes may peel, and there may be a skin rash in the groin area. A low red blood cell count (anaemia), resulting in fatigue, can also occur.

⊕ **IF YOU GET TOO MUCH:** Excess riboflavin isn't dangerous because the body excretes any extra in the urine. However, high intakes of this vitamin can turn the urine bright yellow – a harmless but unsettling side effect.

How to take it

▢ **DOSAGE:** *For cataract prevention*: The usual dosage is 25 mg a day. *For rosacea*: Dosages of 40 mg a day are recommended. *For migraines*: Up to 40 mg a day. Many one-a-day vitamins meet the RDA for riboflavin; high-potency multivitamins may contain much higher amounts – 30 mg or more.

◉ **GUIDELINES FOR USE:** Consult your doctor if you are taking oral contraceptives, antibiotics or psychiatric drugs, which can affect riboflavin needs. Don't take it with alcohol, which reduces absorption of riboflavin in the digestive tract.

Other sources

Good sources of riboflavin include milk, cheese, yoghurt, liver, beef, fish, wholegrain breads and cereals, eggs, avocados and mushrooms.

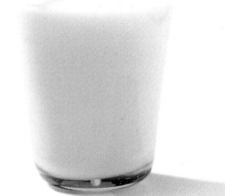

St John's wort

Hypericum perforatum

The ancient Greeks and Romans believed that St John's wort could deter evil spirits. Today the herb has found new and widespread popularity as a natural antidepressant. It is a gentler alternative to conventional medications, with far fewer side effects.

Common uses

- Treats depression.
- Helps to fight off viral and bacterial infections.
- May help to treat PMS, chronic fatigue syndrome and fibromyalgia.
- Helps to relieve chronic pain.
- Soothes haemorrhoids.
- May aid in weight loss.

Forms

- Capsule
- Cream/ointment
- Softgel
- Tablet
- Tincture

CAUTION!

- If you are taking conventional antidepressant drugs, consult your doctor before adding or switching to St John's wort.

- Stop taking St John's wort if you develop a rash, allergy or headaches; seek medical help if you have breathing difficulties.

REMINDER: If you have a medical or psychiatric condition, consult your doctor before taking supplements.

What it is

A shrubby perennial bearing bright yellow flowers, St John's wort is cultivated worldwide. It was named after St John the Baptist because it blooms around 24 June, the day celebrated as his birthday; 'wort' is an old English word for plant. For centuries St John's wort was used to soothe the nerves and to heal wounds and burns. Supplements are made from the dried flowers, which contain a number of therapeutic substances including a healing pigment called hypericin and the chemical hyperforin.

What it does

St John's wort is most frequently used to treat mild depression. Scientists are not sure exactly how the herb works, although it is believed to improve mood and emotions by enhancing brain levels of at least four neurotransmitters, including serotonin.

✪ **MAJOR BENEFITS:** A recent analysis of 23 different studies of St John's wort concluded that the herb was as effective as antidepressant drugs – and more effective than a placebo – in the treatment of mild to moderate depression. (Few studies have examined its usefulness for more serious depression, though it may prove beneficial for this as well.)

St John's wort may be helpful for many conditions associated with depression too, such as anxiety, stress, premenstrual syndrome (PMS), chronic fatigue syndrome, fibromyalgia or chronic pain; it may even have some direct pain-relieving effects. This herb promotes sound sleep and may be especially valuable when depression is marked by fatigue, sleepiness and low energy levels. It may also aid in treating 'wintertime blues' (seasonal affective disorder, or SAD), a type of depression that develops in the autumn and winter and dissipates in the bright sunlight of spring and summer. Some people are wary of

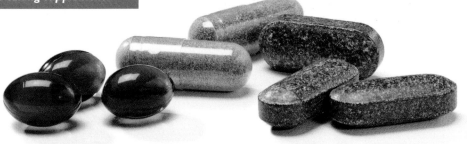

Whether you take softgels, capsules or tablets, St John's wort offers an effective natural remedy for depression.

conventional antidepressants because of their potential for causing undesirable side effects, especially reduced sexual function. St John's wort has far fewer bothersome side effects than these drugs. In addition St John's wort doesn't appear to interact with most other conventional drugs, making it useful for older people taking multiple medications. The herb seems so promising that the US National Institute of Health (NIH) is conducting a major study of its effectiveness.

✦ **ADDITIONAL BENEFITS:** St John's wort fights bacteria and viruses as well. Research indicates that it may play a key part in combating herpes simplex, influenza and Epstein-Barr virus (the cause of glandular fever), and preliminary laboratory studies reveal a possible role for the herb in the fight against AIDS. It also improves liver function. When an ointment made from St John's wort is applied to haemorrhoids it relieves burning and itching. St John's wort may also be useful as a weight-loss aid.

How to take it

✦ **DOSAGE:** The recommended dose is 300 mg of an extract standardised to contain 0.3% hypericin, three times a day. Supplements containing 900 mcg hypericin are also available and can be taken once a day.

✦ **GUIDELINES FOR USE:** Take St John's wort close to mealtime to reduce stomach irritation. In the past, people using the herb were advised not to eat certain foods, including matured cheese and red wine – the same foods best avoided by those taking MAO inhibitors (a treatment for depression). But recent studies suggest that these foods do not present a problem for those on St John's wort.

Like a prescription antidepressant, the herb must build up in your body's tissues before it becomes effective, so be sure to allow at least four weeks to determine whether it works for you. It can be used long term, as needed. Always consult your doctor before taking prescribed antidepressants and St John's wort together. Although adverse reactions are extremely unlikely, it is difficult to evaluate your progress unless the doctor is aware of all the medicines you are taking.

Though no adverse effects have been reported in pregnant or breast-feeding women using the herb, there have been few studies in this group of patients, so caution is advised.

Possible side effects

While uncommon, side effects can include constipation, upset stomach, fatigue, dry mouth and dizziness. People with fair skins are advised to avoid prolonged exposure to sunlight while taking St John's wort. High doses of St John's wort (more than 900 mcg hypericin daily) reduce blood levels of several drugs. If you are taking prescribed medicines, consult your doctor before using this herb. In the Republic of Ireland, St John's wort is now classified as a prescribed medicine.

RECENT FINDINGS

In one recent study 50 people with depression were given either St John's wort or a placebo. After eight weeks 70% of those on St John's wort extract showed marked improvement, as against 45% of those receiving a placebo. No adverse reactions to the herb were noted.

～～～

Several recent trials have compared St John's wort with conventional antidepressants in mild to moderate depression. In one study, 240 people were given either St John's wort or Prozac, and two studies tested St John's wort against imipramine. All three trials found that St John's wort was as effective as conventional antidepressants.

DID YOU KNOW?

In Germany, where doctors routinely prescribe herbal remedies, St John's wort is the most common form of antidepressant – and much more popular than conventional drugs such as Prozac and Zoloft.

Saw palmetto

Serenoa repens

Native Americans regularly consumed the leaf of this small palm tree as a food, so they were probably not plagued by prostate problems. Now frequently prescribed by doctors in Europe, saw palmetto is a herb with men's troubles in mind.

Common uses

- Eases frequent night-time urination and other symptoms of an enlarged prostate.
- Relieves prostate inflammation.
- May boost immunity and treat urinary tract infections.

Forms

- Capsule
- Dried herb/tea
- Softgel
- Tablet
- Tincture

CAUTION!

- Anyone finding blood in the urine or having trouble urinating should see their doctor before taking saw palmetto. These symptoms could be related to prostate cancer.

- Saw palmetto affects hormone levels, so men with prostate cancer and anyone taking hormones should discuss use of the herb with their doctor.

REMINDER: If you have a medical condition, consult your doctor before taking supplements.

What it is

The saw palmetto, a small palm tree that grows wild in the southern USA, gets its name from the spiny saw-toothed stems that lie at the base of each leaf. With a life span of 700 years the plant seems almost indestructible, resisting drought, insect infestation and fire. Its medicinal properties are derived from the blue-black berries, which are usually harvested in August and September. This process is sometimes hazardous: harvesters can easily be cut by the razor-sharp leaf stems, and they risk being bitten by the diamondback rattlesnakes that make their homes in the shade of this scrubby palm.

What it does

Saw palmetto has a long history of folk use. Native Americans valued it for treating disorders of the urinary tract. Early colonists, noting the vitality of animals who fed on the berries, gave the fruits to frail people as a general tonic. Through the years it has also been employed to relieve persistent coughs and improve digestion. Today saw palmetto's claim to fame rests mainly on its ability to relieve the symptoms of an enlarged prostate gland – a use verified by a number of scientific studies.

✦ **MAJOR BENEFITS:** In Italy, Germany, France and other countries, doctors routinely prescribe saw palmetto for the benign (noncancerous) enlargement of the prostate known medically as BPH, which stands for 'benign prostatic hyperplasia', or 'hypertrophy'. When the walnut-sized prostate gland becomes enlarged, a common condition that affects more than half of men over age 50, it can press on the urethra, the tube that carries urine from the bladder through the prostate and out through the penis. The resulting symptoms include frequent urination (especially at

The dried fruit of the saw palmetto tree, often processed into tablets, provides a potent remedy for prostate complaints.

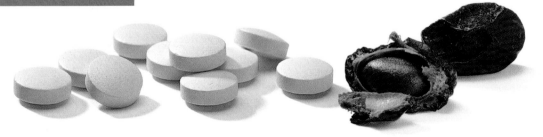

night), weak urine flow, painful urination and difficulty emptying the bladder completely. Researchers believe that saw palmetto relieves the symptoms of BPH in various ways. Most importantly, it appears to alter levels of various hormones that cause prostate cells to multiply. In addition the herb may curb inflammation and reduce tissue swelling.

Studies have found that saw palmetto produces fewer side effects (such as impotence) and quicker results than the conventional prostate drug finasteride (Proscar); it takes only about 30 days to be effective, compared with at least six months for the prescription medication.

☑ **ADDITIONAL BENEFITS:** Although there is strong evidence that saw palmetto relieves the symptoms of BPH, other potential benefits of this herb are more speculative. Saw palmetto has been used to treat certain inflammations of the prostate (prostatitis). In the laboratory it boosts the immune system's ability to kill bacteria, which suggests that it may be a potential treatment for prostate or urinary tract infections. Saw palmetto affects levels of cancer-promoting hormones, so scientists are also investigating its possible role in preventing prostate cancer.

How to take it

☑ **DOSAGE:** The usual dosage is 160 mg twice a day. Be careful about taking higher amounts: scientific studies have not examined the effects of daily doses above 320 mg. Choose supplements made from extracts standardised to contain 85% to 95% fatty acids and sterols – the active ingredients in the berries that are responsible for its therapeutic effects.

◈ **GUIDELINES FOR USE:** Since prostatic enlargement could be a result of cancer, you must obtain a correct diagnosis before taking this herb to treat BPH. Also consult your doctor before taking saw palmetto for prostatitis. Saw palmetto has a bitter taste, so those using the liquid form may want to dilute it in a small amount of water. The herb can be taken with or without food. Although some healers recommend sipping tea made from saw palmetto, it may not contain therapeutic amounts of the active ingredients – and so provide few benefits for the treatment of BPH.

Possible side effects

Side effects are relatively uncommon, but include mild abdominal pain, nausea, dizziness and headache. If side effects occur, lower the dose or stop taking the herb.

RECENT FINDINGS

In an international study of 1000 men with moderate BPH, two-thirds benefited from taking either a prescription prostate drug (Proscar) or saw palmetto for six months. Those using the herb had fewer problems with side effects linked with the drug, such as reduced libido and impotence. However, the drug significantly reduced the size of the prostate, whereas the effect of saw palmetto was much less dramatic, particularly in men with very large prostates. The study's authors concluded that the herb may be most useful when the gland is only slightly or moderately enlarged.

Selenium

Although the significance of this trace mineral was not widely acknowledged until 1979, selenium has now gained prominence as a potentially powerful weapon against cancer. Many researchers believe that it could prove to be one of the most important disease-fighting nutrients.

Common uses

- *Works with vitamin E to help to prevent cancer and heart disease.*
- *Protects against cataracts and macular degeneration.*
- *Fights viral infections; reduces the severity of cold sores and shingles; may slow down the development of HIV/AIDS.*
- *Helps to relieve lupus symptoms.*

Forms

- Capsule
- Tablet

What it is

A trace mineral essential for many body processes, selenium is found in soil. The mineral is present throughout the body but is most abundant in the kidneys, liver, spleen, pancreas and testes.

What it does

Selenium acts as an antioxidant, blocking the rogue molecules known as free radicals that damage DNA. It is part of an antioxidant enzyme (called glutathione peroxidase) that protects cells against environmental and dietary toxins, and is often included with vitamins C and E in antioxidant 'cocktails'. This combination may guard against a range of disorders thought to be caused by free-radical damage – from cancer, heart disease and strokes to cataracts and macular degeneration.

✪ **MAJOR BENEFITS:** Selenium has received a great deal of attention for its role in combating cancer. A five-year US study, conducted at Cornell University and the University of Arizona, showed that taking 200 mcg of selenium daily resulted in 63% fewer prostate tumours, 58% fewer colo-rectal cancers, 46% fewer lung malignancies and a 39% overall decrease cancer. deaths. In other studies, selenium showed promise in preventing cancers of the ovaries, cervix, rectum, bladder, oesophagus, pancreas and liver, as well as leukaemia. Studies of cancer patients reveal that people with the lowest blood levels of selenium developed more tumours and had a higher rate of disease recurrence, a greater risk of cancer spreading and a shorter overall survival rate than those with high selenium levels.

In addition, selenium can protect the heart, primarily by reducing the 'stickiness' of the blood and decreasing the risk of clotting, which in turn lowers the risk of heart attack and stroke. Selenium increases the ratio of HDL ('good') cholesterol to LDL ('bad') cholesterol, which is critical for a healthy heart. Smokers and anyone who has already had a heart attack or stroke may gain the greatest cardiovascular benefits from selenium supplements, though everyone may profit from taking selenium in a daily vitamin and mineral supplement.

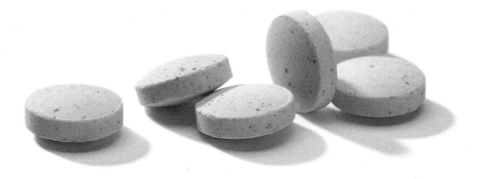

❋ ADDITIONAL BENEFITS: Selenium may be useful in preventing cataracts and macular degeneration, the leading causes of impaired vision or blindness in the elderly. It is also vital for converting thyroid hormone, which is needed for the proper functioning of every cell in the body, from a less active form (called T4) to its active form (known as T3). In addition, selenium is essential for a healthy immune system, assisting the body in defending itself against harmful bacteria and viruses as well as cancer cells. Its immunity-boosting effects may play a role in fighting the herpes virus that is responsible for cold sores and shingles, and it is also being studied for possible effectiveness against HIV, the virus that causes AIDS.

When combined with vitamin E, selenium appears to have some anti-inflammatory benefits as well. These two nutrients may improve chronic conditions such as rheumatoid arthritis, psoriasis, lupus and eczema.

How much you need

The recommended target intake for selenium is 75 mcg for men and 60 mcg for women daily. However, a therapeutic dose of up to 200 mcg a day may be needed to produce major benefits.

⊟ IF YOU GET TOO LITTLE: Soil with low levels of selenium, such as in the UK, produces food containing relatively low levels of the nutrient. Consistent intakes below the recommended amount could lead to higher incidences of cancer, heart disease, immune problems and inflammatory conditions of all kinds, particularly those affecting the skin. Insufficient amounts of selenium during pregnancy could increase the risk of birth defects (especially those involving the heart) or, possibly, sudden infant death syndrome (SIDS). Early symptoms of selenium deficiency include muscular weakness and fatigue.

⊞ IF YOU GET TOO MUCH: It is hard to get too much selenium from your diet, but if you are taking this mineral in supplement form it is important to remember that the margin of safety between a therapeutic dose of selenium (up to 350 mcg a day) and a toxic dose (as little as 900 mcg) is small compared with that of other nutrients. Symptoms of toxicity include nervousness, depression, nausea and vomiting, a garlicky odour to the breath and perspiration, and a loss of hair and fingernails.

How to take it

⊘ DOSAGE: Most nutritionists agree that the optimum dose for long-term use of selenium should be between 100 and 200 mcg daily.

◉ GUIDELINES FOR USE: Vitamin E greatly enhances the effectiveness of selenium; people at risk of heart disease may wish to add foods rich in this vitamin to their diet.

Other sources

The most abundant sources of selenium include Brazil nuts, seafood, poultry and meats. Grains, particularly oats and brown rice, may also have significant amounts, depending on the selenium content of the soil in which they were grown.

RECENT FINDINGS

Recent studies show that in the test tube selenium works relatively quickly, helping cells to grow and die at normal rates and protecting them from becoming cancerous. Researchers believe that selenium's cancer-fighting benefits may be fast-acting in the body as well.

Studies in mice show that a deficiency in either selenium or vitamin E – both antioxidants – can convert a latent, inactive virus into its active, disease-causing form. This may help to explain why selenium is effective against cold sores and shingles, which are both caused by reactivation of a dormant herpes virus.

DID YOU KNOW?

Brazil nuts are very rich in selenium; one nut may contain about 75 mcg, the recommended daily target for a man. Kidneys are also an excellent source of selenium; a single lamb's kidney contains about 50 mcg.

Tea tree oil

Melaleuca alternifolia

For centuries aboriginal Australians relied on the leaves of the tea tree to fight infections. Today tea tree oil is valued throughout the world as a potent antiseptic, and scientists have confirmed its powerful ability to combat harmful bacteria and fungal infections.

Common uses

- *Disinfects and promotes the healing of cuts and scrapes.*
- *Minimises scarring.*
- *Speeds recovery from insect bites and stings, including bee stings.*
- *Fights athlete's foot, fungal nail infections and yeast infections.*

Forms

- Cream
- Gel
- Oil
- Vaginal suppository

CAUTION!

- Tea tree oil is for topical use only. Do not ingest; it can be toxic. Keep it away from eyes.

- Consult your doctor before applying to deep open wounds.

REMINDER: If you have a medical condition, consult your doctor before taking supplements.

What it is

A champion infection fighter, tea tree oil has a pleasant nutmeg-like scent. It comes from the leaves of *Melaleuca alternifolia*, or the tea tree, a species that grows only in Australia (and is completely different from the species of *Camellia* used to make black, oolong and green drinking teas). Extracted through a steam-distillation process, quality tea tree oil contains at least 40% terpinen-4-ol – the active ingredient responsible for its healing effects – and less than 5% cineole, a substance that causes skin irritation if too much is present. With the rise of antibiotics after the Second World War, tea tree oil fell out of favour. Recently interest in it has revived, and more than 700 tonnes are now produced annually.

What it does

Tea tree oil is used topically to treat a variety of common infections. Once applied to the skin, the oil makes it impossible for many disease-causing fungi to survive. Studies have shown that it also fights various bacteria, including some that are resistant to powerful antibiotics. Doctors think that one reason why tea tree oil is so effective is that it readily mixes with skin oils, allowing it to attack the infective agent quickly and actively.

MAJOR BENEFITS: Tea tree oil's antiseptic properties are especially useful for treating cuts and scrapes, as well as insect bites and stings. The oil promotes the healing of minor wounds, helps to prevent infection and minimises any future scarring. As an antifungal agent, tea tree oil fights the fungus *Trichophyton*, the culprit in athlete's foot, a similar infection of the groin and some nail infections. It may also be effective against *Candida albicans* and *Tricho-monas vaginalis*, two of the organisms that cause vaginal infections. Some fungal infections can be stubborn to treat, however, and your doctor may need to prescribe a more potent conventional antifungal medication.

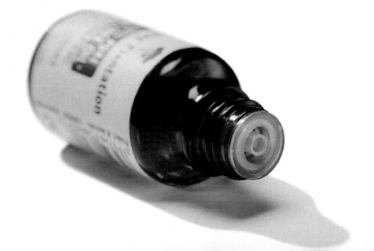

✣ **ADDITIONAL BENEFITS:** Tea tree oil may be beneficial in the treatment of acne. In one study, a gel containing 5% tea tree oil was shown to be as effective against acne as a lotion with 5% benzoyl peroxide, the active ingredient in most over-the-counter acne medications. But there were fewer side effects with tea tree oil: it caused less scaling, dryness and itching than the benzoyl peroxide formula. Another study found that a solution containing 0.5% tea tree oil offered protection against *Pityrosporum ovale*, a common dandruff-causing fungus. Sometimes tea tree oil is suggested as a treatment for warts, which are caused by viruses, though studies have not confirmed its efficacy in this respect.

How to take it

✐ **DOSAGE:** *To treat athlete's foot, skin wounds or nail infections*: Apply a drop or two of pure, undiluted tea tree oil to affected areas of the skin or nails two or three times a day. Tea tree oil creams and lotions can also be used. *To treat vaginal yeast infections*: Insert a commercially available tea tree oil vaginal suppository every 12 hours, for up to five days.

◐ **GUIDELINES FOR USE:** Tea tree oil is for topical use only. Never take tea tree oil orally. If you ingest it, or a child does, phone your doctor or get to a hospital casualty department immediately. Rarely, tea tree oil can cause an allergic skin rash in some people. Before using the oil for the first time, dab a small amount on your inner arm with a cotton swab. If you are allergic, your arm will quickly become red or inflamed. If this response occurs, dilute the oil by adding a few drops to a tablespoon of bland oil, such as vegetable oil or almond oil, and try the arm test again. If you have no skin reaction it is safe to apply the diluted oil elsewhere.

Possible side effects

Although tea tree oil can cause minor skin irritation, it otherwise appears to be safe for topical use. Like many herbal oils in pure, undiluted form, it can irritate the eyes and mucous membranes.

Tea tree oil is often added to soaps and skin-care products because of its ability to destroy bacteria.

BUYING GUIDE

■ A number of shampoos, soaps and other skin-care products contain tea tree oil, but many have such a small amount that they have little or no bacteria-fighting effect. Contact the manufacturer to find out if any studies on a product's effectiveness have been conducted.

■ There is more than one type of tea tree, so when buying tea tree oil check that it is derived from *Melaleuca alternifolia*. Oil from other species tends to be high in cineole content and does not have the same medicinal properties.

RECENT FINDINGS

In one recent test-tube study, tea tree oil (as well as peppermint, cinnamon leaf and nutmeg oils) was reported to contain substances that are toxic to head lice. Additional study is needed on people before tea tree oil can be recommended to combat lice, particularly in children, who may be especially sensitive to this oil.

Swiss researchers found that a special medical preparation of tea tree oil offers protection against cavity-forming bacteria in the mouth. But never use the pure oil in your mouth; it can be irritating and is dangerous if swallowed. Tea tree toothpastes are probably safe because they have so little oil – but, for the same reason, they may have limited bacteria-fighting benefits.

Thiamin

Most of us get enough thiamin in our diets to meet our basic needs, but many nutritionists believe that some people, especially older adults, are mildly deficient in this B vitamin, which makes a vital contribution to a healthy metabolism and a properly functioning nervous system.

Common uses

- Aids energy production.
- Promotes healthy nerves.
- May improve mood.
- Strengthens the heart.
- Soothes indigestion.

Forms

- Capsule
- Tablet

What it is

Thiamin, an often overlooked but key member of the B-complex vitamin family, is known as vitamin B_1 because it was the first B vitamin to be discovered. Although severe thiamin deficiency is a thing of the past, even a moderate deficit has health consequences. Thiamin is available as an individual supplement, but it is advisable to get it from a B-complex supplement because it works closely with the other B vitamins.

What it does

Thiamin is essential for converting the carbohydrates in foods into energy. It also promotes healthy nerves and may be useful in treating certain types of heart disease.

MAJOR BENEFITS: In people with heart disease, thiamin can improve the pumping power of the heart. Thiamin levels in the body are depleted by long-term treatment with diuretic drugs, which are often prescribed for heart patients to reduce the fluid build-up associated with the disease. In one study, patients with heart disease who took furosemide (a diuretic) were given either 200 mg a day of thiamin or a placebo. After six weeks, the thiamin group showed a 22% improvement.

By helping to maintain healthy nerves, thiamin may minimise tingling and numbness in the hands and feet, a problem that frequently plagues people with diabetes or other diseases that cause nerve damage.

ADDITIONAL BENEFITS: In combination with choline and pantothenic acid (also B vitamins), thiamin can enhance the digestive process and provide relief from indigestion. Some researchers think that a thiamin deficiency is linked to mental illnesses, including depression, and that high-dose thiamin supplementation may be beneficial.

Thiamin may also help to boost memory in people with Alzheimer's disease – but evidence is far from conclusive. However, the confusion that is common in older adults after surgery may be prevented by

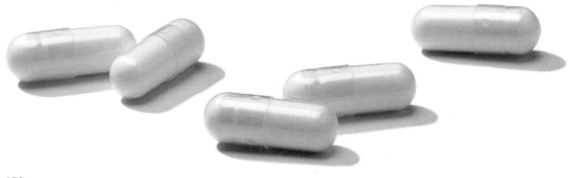

additional doses of thiamin in the weeks before an operation. Doctors also use thiamin to treat the psychosis related to alcohol withdrawal. Antiseizure medications interfere with the vitamin's absorption, so people taking them may need extra thiamin; this may also reduce the fuzzy thinking that such drugs can cause.

How much you need

The recommended amount of 1 mg a day for men and 0.8 mg a day for women is enough to maintain good health and to prevent a thiamin deficiency. However, higher doses are recommended for therapeutic use.

⊟ **IF YOU GET TOO LITTLE:** A mild thiamin deficiency may go unnoticed. Its symptoms are irritability, depression, muscle weakness and weight loss. A severe thiamin deficiency causes beriberi, a disease that leads to mental impairment, the wasting away of muscle, paralysis, nerve damage and eventually death. Once rampant in many countries, beriberi is rare today. It is seen only in parts of Asia where the diet consists mainly of white rice, which is stripped of thiamin and other nutrients during milling. In the UK, thiamin is added to white flour and many breakfast cereals.

⊞ **IF YOU GET TOO MUCH:** There are no adverse effects associated with high doses of thiamin, because the body is efficient at eliminating excess amounts through the urine.

How to take it

▨ **DOSAGE:** Specific disorders can benefit from supplemental thiamin. *For heart disease*: Take 50 mg of thiamin daily. *For numbness and tingling*: Take 50 mg of thiamin a day, preferably as part of a B-complex supplement. *For depression*: Take 50 mg daily as part of a B-complex supplement. *For indigestion*: Take 50 mg a day in the morning. *For alcoholism*: Take 50 mg daily, preferably as part of a B-complex supplement.

◉ **GUIDELINES FOR USE:** Thiamin is best absorbed in an acidic environment. Take it with meals, when stomach acid is produced to digest food. Divide your dose in half and take the halves at different times of the day; high doses are readily flushed out of the body in urine.

Other sources

Lean pork is probably the best dietary source of thiamin, followed by whole grains, dried beans and nuts and seeds. Enriched grain products also contain thiamin.

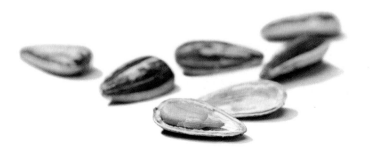

Turmeric

Curcuma longa

A main ingredient of curry powder, turmeric has been used in Indian and Chinese medicine for thousands of years to relieve conditions ranging from flatulence to menstrual irregularities. It is now recognised in the West as a powerful antioxidant and anti-inflammatory agent.

Common uses

- *Reduces inflammation, especially in shoulder, knee and elbow joints.*
- *Can relieve the inflammation and pain of rheumatoid arthritis.*
- *May lower cholesterol levels and reduce tendency to thrombosis.*
- *May help to prevent cancer, particularly of the colon and mouth.*

Forms

- Capsule
- Powder
- Tablet

CAUTION!

- **Do not exceed the recommended dose. Although generally safe, turmeric in large doses may cause gastrointestinal problems or even ulcers.**

REMINDER: If you have a medical condition, consult your doctor before taking supplements.

What it is

The yellow-flowered turmeric plant is a member of the ginger family. It is grown in Indonesia, China, India and other parts of the tropics, where the dried aromatic root-like stem is ground to form a powder. It contains yellow-coloured curcumin, the key active component, and also an orange-coloured volatile oil. The herb has been shown to have a positive effect on a variety of medical conditions.

Apart from its culinary uses, turmeric is used as a preservative, colorant and flavouring agent in many food products including baked foods, pickles and meat products.

What it does

Turmeric has an antioxidant effect approximately equivalent to that of Vitamins C and E, meaning that it provides powerful protection against the damage that can be done to the cells of the body by unstable oxygen molecules called free radicals. Turmeric, and especially its component curcumin, acts as an anti-inflammatory agent both when applied topically as a poultice and when used orally. Laboratory studies suggest that turmeric may have significant anticarcinogenic properties, and animal studies indicate that it may lower blood cholesterol levels. Its anti-inflammatory and antioxidant properties, combined with its ability to increase the secretion of bile and the production of liver enzymes, explains its liver-protective effects against toxins.

MAJOR BENEFITS: If turmeric is taken internally its principal effects are associated with the ability of curcumin to suppress the release of

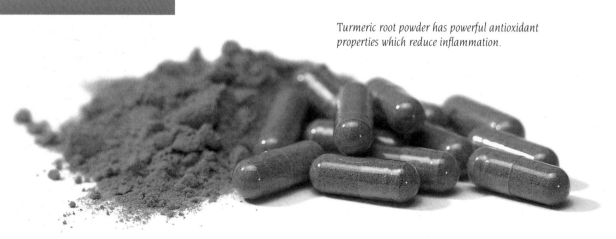

Turmeric root powder has powerful antioxidant properties which reduce inflammation.

inflammatory agents within the body's tissues. It is also thought to stimulate the production of cortisone from the adrenal glands, which indirectly assists the healing process.

Curcumin has been shown in animal studies to have therapeutic properties equivalent to those of cortisone and phenylbutazone in cases of acute inflammation (although it is only half as effective in chronic cases), with the advantage that it has no toxic results. If turmeric is applied to the skin, as is common in India, it can ease pain and inflammation in muscles and joints. Laboratory research has shown that turmeric can not only inhibit the early development of cancer cells but may also stop the progression of the disease as well as boosting the body's own antioxidant system. By lowering cholesterol levels and preventing the coagulation of blood platelets, turmeric has a role to play in combating atherosclerosis, even when taken in small doses.

Its combination of antioxidant and anti-inflammatory properties, together with its ability to increase bile acid output, provides evidence to support the traditional use of turmeric for protecting the liver. A preliminary study has shown the herb to be helpful for people with indigestion. By both hindering the formation of wind and releasing it if it does form, turmeric has a positive effect on the gastrointestinal system and can also inhibit intestinal spasm.

⊛ **ADDITIONAL BENEFITS:** In a clinical trial, patients suffering from rheumatoid arthritis were given 1200 mg of curcumin a day and the results were compared with those of a group given the traditional treatment of 300 mg of phenylbutazone. Both groups reported similar improvements in walking time, stiffness and joint swelling, and, unlike phenylbutazone, curcumin has no adverse side effects when taken in the correct amounts.

How to take it

⊘ **DOSAGE:** The recommended dose for turmeric is between 500 mg and 1000 mg of the dried standardised root extract (containing 95% curcuminoids) per day. As an anti-inflammatory: Take 300 mg up to three times a day with meals.

⊙ **GUIDELINES FOR USE:** If turmeric is combined with the enzyme bromelain to improve absorption, it should be taken between meals for best results.

Possible side effects

Turmeric appears to be very safe in recommended doses. However, there is some evidence to suggest that – because turmeric enhances the release of bile in the liver – high doses should not be taken by people with gallstones, since gallstones can hinder the flow of bile.

BUYING GUIDE

■ When you are buying a turmeric supplement ensure that it is a standardised root extract containing 95% curcuminoids.

RECENT FINDINGS

In one trial 62 patients with ulcerating mouth or skin tumours which had not responded to traditional treatments such as chemotherapy, radiotherapy or surgery were treated with an external application of turmeric extract or curcumin three times a day for 18 months. At the end of the study it was found that itching had been reduced by 70%, pain by 50% and the size of the lesion by 10%.

DID YOU KNOW?

Turmeric's name comes from the Latin *terra merita*, meaning 'meritorious earth'. This may have been an early reference to the plant's many beneficial properties.

FACTS & TIPS

■ Increasing the turmeric intake in your diet may be beneficial in some cases, but it would be necessary to consume large quantities to obtain the amount required for a specific medical effect.

■ There is no evidence that turmeric has irritant effects when taken in recommended amounts. Indeed, it may provide protection against the formation of ulcers.

Valerian

Valeriana officinalis

It is three o'clock in the morning and you are wide awake – again. You wish there was something that you could safely take to induce temporary oblivion. Valerian may be the answer: this herb gently encourages sleep without the unpleasant side effects of conventional drugs.

Common uses

- *Promotes restful sleep.*
- *Soothes stress and anxiety.*
- *Improves the symptoms of some digestive disorders.*

Forms

- Capsule
- Dried herb/tea
- Softgel
- Tablet
- Tincture

What it is

In the UK, Germany and other European countries, valerian is officially approved as a sleep aid by medical authorities. A perennial plant native to North America and Europe, valerian has pinkish-coloured flowers that grow from a tuberous rootstock, or rhizome. Harvested when the plant is two years old, the rootstock contains a number of important compounds – valepotriates, valeric acid and volatile oils among them – that at one time or another were each thought to be responsible for the herb's sedative powers. Many herbalists believe that valerian's effectiveness may be the result of synergy among the various compounds.

What it does

Taken for centuries as an aid to sleep, valerian can also act as a calming agent in stressful daytime situations. It is used in treating anxiety disorders and conditions worsened by stress, such as diverticular disorders and irritable bowel syndrome.

⊛ **MAJOR BENEFITS:** Compounds in valerian are able to raise levels in the brain of a nerve chemical (neurotransmitter) called gamma-aminobutyric acid, or GABA. It is through this interaction that valerian promotes sleep and eases anxiety. Unlike benzodiazepines – drugs such as diazepam (Valium) or alprazolam (Xanax), commonly prescribed for these disorders – valerian is not addictive and does not make you feel drugged. Rather than inducing sleep directly, valerian calms the brain and body so sleep

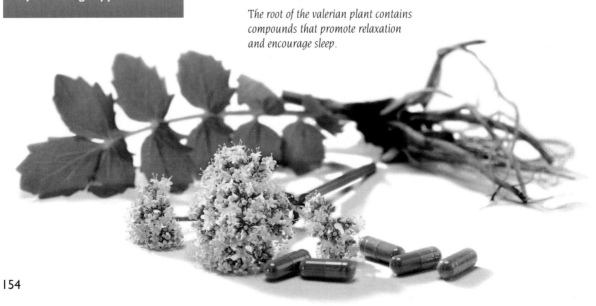

The root of the valerian plant contains compounds that promote relaxation and encourage sleep.

can occur naturally. One of the benefits of valerian for insomniacs is that, when taken at recommended doses, it doesn't make you feel groggy in the morning as some prescription drugs do.

According to various studies, valerian works as well as prescription drugs for many individuals, and when compared with a placebo, appears to lull a person to sleep. In one study, 128 people were given one of two valerian preparations or a placebo. It was found that the herb improved sleep quality: those taking valerian fell asleep more quickly and woke up less often than those receiving a placebo. In another study involving insomniacs, nearly all reported improved sleep when taking valerian, and 44% classified their sleep quality as perfect.

Although modern interest in valerian as an aid against anxiety is relatively recent, the herb is increasingly recommended by herbalists for this purpose.

ADDITIONAL BENEFITS: Valerian helps to relax the smooth muscle of the gastrointestinal tract, making it valuable for the treatment of irritable bowel syndrome and diverticular disorders, which often involve painful spasms of the intestine. In addition, because flare-ups of these disorders are sometimes triggered by stress, valerian's calming action may also account for its effectiveness.

How to take it

DOSAGE: *For insomnia*: Take 250 to 500 mg of the powdered extract in capsule or tablet form or 1 teaspoon of the tincture 30 to 45 minutes before bedtime. Studies show that, for most people, higher doses bring no additional benefit. However, if the low dose does not work for you, you can safely use as much as 900 mg (2 teaspoons of the tincture). *For anxiety*: Consume 250 mg twice a day and 250 to 500 mg prior to bedtime.

GUIDELINES FOR USE: Valerian has a slightly unpleasant taste, so if you choose the tincture try blending it with a little honey or sugar to make it more palatable. Although valerian is not addictive, it is inadvisable to rely on any substance, herbal or otherwise, to help you to fall asleep each night. Therefore, avoid taking valerian nightly for more than two weeks in a row, and ensure that you do not combine it with prescription sleeping drugs or tranquillisers. It is safe to take valerian with other herbs, such as chamomile, melissa (also known as lemon balm) or passionflower, which may increase its effectiveness as a sleeping aid. Valerian can also be used with St John's wort if you are feeling depressed.

Possible side effects

Studies have shown that, even in amounts 20 times higher than normally recommended, valerian has no dangerous side effects. However, extremely large doses can cause dizziness, restlessness, blurred vision, nausea, headache, giddiness and grogginess in the morning.

BUYING GUIDE

When buying valerian, look for a product which is a 5:1 herb extract ratio.

RECENT FINDINGS

Prescription sleeping drugs often cause grogginess the morning after they are taken and can impair a person's ability to drive or to perform other tasks that require concentration. Valerian does not, according to a German study. Researchers compared the effects of valerian, valerian and hops, a benzodiazepine drug and a placebo. The herbal preparations and the drug all improved sleep quality. The benzodiazepine drug reduced performance the following morning, but the herbs did not.

DID YOU KNOW?

Valerian preparations have a very disagreeable odour – so much so that inexperienced users may think they have a bad batch. Don't be put off by the smell; it's quite normal.

Vitamin A

This essential nutrient keeps the eyesight keen, the skin healthy and the immune system strong. Consequently the body needs adequate levels of vitamin A to ensure the prevention of various eye problems, a number of skin disorders and a wide range of infections.

Common uses

- Helps the body to fight colds, flu and other types of infections.
- Promotes skin health and healing of wounds, burns and ulcers.
- Maintains healthy eyes.
- Benefits the lining of the digestive tract.

Forms

- Capsule
- Liquid
- Softgel
- Tablet

What it is

Vitamin A, a fat-soluble nutrient, is stored in the liver. The body gets part of its vitamin A from animal fats and makes part in the intestine from beta-carotene and other carotenoids in fruit and vegetables. Vitamin A is present in the body in various chemical forms called retinoids – so named because the vitamin is essential to the health of the retina.

What it does

This vitamin prevents night blindness, maintains the skin and cells that line the respiratory and gastrointestinal tracts and helps to build teeth and bones. It is vital for normal reproduction, growth and development. In addition, vitamin A is crucial to the immune system, including the plentiful supply of immune cells that line the airways and digestive tract and form an important line of defence against disease.

MAJOR BENEFITS: Vitamin A is perhaps best known for its ability to maintain vision, especially night vision, assisting the eye in adjusting from bright light to darkness. It can also alleviate 'dry eye', a complaint which is common in many developing countries and is specifically associated with severe vitamin A deficiency.

By boosting immunity, vitamin A greatly strengthens resistance to infections, including sore throat, colds, flu and bronchitis. It may also combat cold sores and shingles (caused by a herpes virus), warts (a viral skin infection), eye infections and vaginal yeast infections – and perhaps even help to control allergies. The vitamin may help the immune system to battle against breast and lung cancers and improve survival rates in those with leukaemia; in addition, animal studies suggest it inhibits melanoma, a deadly form of skin cancer. Another benefit for cancer patients is that the effectiveness of chemotherapy may be enhanced when the body has good levels of vitamin A.

ADDITIONAL BENEFITS: Vitamin A was first used in the 1940s to treat skin disorders, including acne and psoriasis, but the doses were high and toxic. Scientists later developed safer vitamin A derivatives (notably retinoic acid); now sold as prescription drugs, these include the acne and antiwrinkle cream Retin-A. Lower doses of vitamin A (7500 mcg a day)

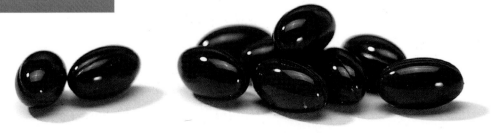

can be used, but only under the supervision of a doctor, to treat a range of skin conditions, including acne, dry skin, eczema, rosacea and psoriasis. When vitamin A levels in the body are good, the healing of skin wounds is promoted, and even recovery from sprains and strains may be hastened. The value of good vitamin A levels even extends to the lining of the digestive tract, where it helps to treat inflammatory bowel disease and ulcers. In addition, getting enough of this vitamin will speed up recovery in people who have had strokes. Women with heavy or prolonged menstrual periods are sometimes deficient in this vitamin.

How much you need

The recommended target for vitamin A is 600 mcg a day for women and 700 mcg a day for men.

⊟ **IF YOU GET TOO LITTLE:** Although quite rare in the UK, a vitamin A deficiency can cause night blindness (even total blindness) and a greatly lowered resistance to infection. Milder cases of deficiency do occur, especially in the elderly, who often have vitamin-poor diets. Infections such as pneumonia can deplete vitamin A stores.

⊞ **IF YOU GET TOO MUCH:** Although levels of up to 1500 mcg a day are safe, supplementation with vitamin A should not be undertaken unless prescribed by a doctor. This advice is particularly important for women who are pregnant or are likely to become pregnant, because of risk of damage to the developing foetus. Above these levels, an overabundance of vitamin A can be a real problem. A single dose of 150,000 mcg may induce weakness and vomiting; and as little as 7500 mcg a day for six years has been reported to cause serious liver disease (cirrhosis). Signs of toxicity include dry, cracking skin and brittle nails, hair that falls out easily, bleeding gums, weight loss, irritability, fatigue and nausea.

How to take it

☑ **DOSAGE:** To avoid an excessive intake of vitamin A it is advisable to take supplements containing no more than the recommended daily allowance of 800 mcg a day. Alternatively, take vitamin A in the form of mixed carotenoids.

◉ **GUIDELINES FOR USE:** Take supplements with food; a little fat in the diet aids absorption. Vitamin E and zinc help the body to use vitamin A, which in turn boosts absorption of iron from foods.

Other sources

Vitamin A is richly represented in fish, egg yolks, butter, offal such as liver (90 grams provide more than 2500 mcg), and fortified milk (check the label to be sure). Yellow, orange, red and dark green fruits and vegetables have large amounts of beta-carotene and many other carotenoids, which the body makes into vitamin A when needed.

Vitamin B₆

The 'workhorse' of nutrients, vitamin B_6 is probably involved in more bodily processes than any other vitamin. Surveys indicate, however, that a fifth of women and the same proportion of elderly people are not obtaining enough of this critically important nutrient from their daily diets.

Common uses

- *Helps to prevent cardiovascular disease and strokes.*
- *Helps to lift depression.*
- *Eases insomnia.*
- *Treats carpal tunnel syndrome.*
- *May lessen PMS symptoms.*
- *Helps to relieve asthma attacks.*

Forms

- Capsule
- Liquid
- Tablet

CAUTION!

- Long-term use of high doses of B_6 may cause nerve damage.

REMINDER: If you have a medical or psychiatric condition, consult your doctor before taking supplements.

What it is

Vitamin B_6 performs more than 100 jobs innumerable times a day. It functions primarily as a coenzyme, a substance that acts in concert with enzymes to speed up chemical reactions in the cells.

Another name for vitamin B_6 is pyridoxine. In supplement form it is available as pyridoxine hydrochloride or pyridoxal-5-phosphate (P-5-P). Either form satisfies most needs, but some nutritionally aware doctors prefer P-5-P because it may be more easily absorbed.

What it does

Forming red blood cells, helping cells to make proteins, manufacturing brain chemicals (neurotransmitters) such as serotonin and releasing stored forms of energy are just a few of the functions of vitamin B_6. There is also evidence to suggest that it plays a role in preventing and treating many diseases.

PREVENTION: Getting enough B_6 through diet or supplements may help to prevent heart disease. Working with folic acid and vitamin B_{12}, this vitamin assists the body in processing homocysteine, an amino acid-like compound that has been linked to an increased risk of heart disease and other vascular disorders when large amounts are present in the blood.

ADDITIONAL BENEFITS: Some women suffering from premenstrual syndrome (PMS) report that vitamin B_6 provides relief from many of the symptoms. This beneficial effect probably occurs as a result of the vitamin's involvement in clearing excess oestrogen from the body. In its role as a building block for neurotransmitters, vitamin B_6 may be useful in reducing the likelihood of epileptic seizures as well as improving the moods of people suffering from depression. In fact, up to 25% of people with depression may be deficient in vitamin B_6.

The vitamin also maintains nerve health. People with diabetes, who are at risk of nerve damage, can also benefit from supplements of vitamin B_6. In addition, it is effective in easing the symptoms of carpal tunnel syndrome, which involves nerve inflammation in the wrist. And for people with asthma, vitamin B_6 may reduce the intensity and frequency of attacks; it is especially important for those taking the asthma drug theophylline.

How much you need

The recommended target for vitamin B_6 is 1.2 mg a day for women and 1.4 mg a day for men. Therapeutic doses are higher.

⊖ **IF YOU GET TOO LITTLE:** A recent survey found that a fifth of all women fail to meet the recommended target for vitamin B_6. Women taking oral contraceptives may have especially low levels of this vitamin. Mild deficiencies of B_6 can raise homocysteine levels, increasing the risk of heart and vascular diseases. Symptoms of severe deficiency, which is rare, are skin disorders such as dermatitis, sores around the mouth and acne. Neurological signs include insomnia, depression and, in extreme cases, seizures and brain wave abnormalities.

⊕ **IF YOU GET TOO MUCH:** High doses of vitamin B_6 (more than 2000 mg a day) can cause nerve damage when taken for long periods. In rare cases, prolonged use at lower doses (more than 200 mg a day) can have the same consequence. Fortunately, nerve damage is completely reversible once you discontinue the vitamin. If you are using vitamin B_6 for nerve pain, contact your doctor if you experience any new numbness or tingling and stop taking the vitamin. Doses up to 10 mg a day are safe for long-term use, but doses of up to 200 mg may be taken for short periods of time.

How to take it

▨ **DOSAGE:** You can keep homocysteine levels in check with just 3 mg of B_6 a day, but a daily dose of 50 mg is often recommended. Higher doses are needed for therapeutic uses. *For PMS:* Take 100 mg of B_6 a day. *For acute carpal tunnel syndrome:* Try 50 mg of B_6 or P-5-P three times a day. *For asthma:* Take 50 mg of B_6 twice a day.

◉ **GUIDELINES FOR USE:** Vitamin B_6 is best absorbed in amounts of no more than 100 mg at one time. When you are taking higher doses this more gradual intake will also decrease your chances of nerve damage.

Other sources

Fish, poultry, meats, chickpeas, potatoes, avocados and bananas are all good sources of vitamin B_6.

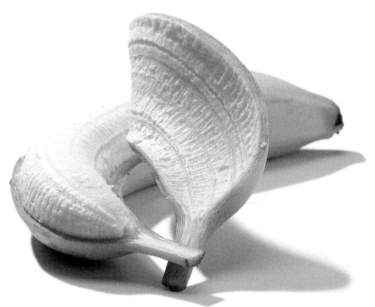

Vitamin B$_{12}$

Although this vitamin is plentiful in most people's diets, after the age of 50 some people have a limited ability to absorb it from food. Supplements may be useful, because even mild deficiencies may increase the risk of heart disease, depression and possibly Alzheimer's disease.

Common uses

- *Prevents a form of anaemia.*
- *Helps to reduce depression.*
- *Thwarts nerve pain, numbness and tingling.*
- *Lowers the risk of heart disease.*
- *May improve multiple sclerosis and tinnitus.*

Forms

- Capsule
- Tablet

CAUTION!

- If you take a vitamin B$_{12}$ supplement you must also have a folic acid supplement: a high intake of one can mask a deficiency of the other.

- Diagnosis of pernicious anaemia should be made by a doctor, and regular follow-up blood tests may be necessary.

REMINDER: If you have a medical or psychiatric condition, consult your doctor before taking supplements.

What it is

Vitamin B$_{12}$, also known as cobalamin, was the most recent vitamin to be discovered. In the late 1940s it was identified as the substance in calves' liver that cured pernicious anaemia, a potentially fatal disease primarily affecting older adults. Vitamin B$_{12}$ is the only B vitamin the body stores in large amounts, mostly in the liver. The body absorbs B$_{12}$ through a very complicated process: digestive enzymes in the presence of enough stomach acid separate B$_{12}$ from the protein in foods. The vitamin then binds with a substance called intrinsic factor (a protein produced by cells in the stomach lining) before being carried to the small intestine, where it is absorbed. Low levels of stomach acid or an inadequate amount of intrinsic factor – both of which occur with age – can lead to deficiencies. However, because the body has good reserves of B$_{12}$, it can take several years for a shortfall to develop.

What it does

Vitamin B$_{12}$ is essential for cell replication and is particularly important for red blood-cell production. It maintains the protective sheath around nerves (myelin), assists in converting food to energy and plays a critical role in the production of DNA and RNA, the genetic material in cells.

PREVENTION: Moderately high blood levels of homocysteine, an amino acid-like substance, have been linked to an increased risk of heart disease. Working with folic acid, vitamin B$_{12}$ helps the body to process homocysteine and so may lower that risk. Vitamin B$_{12}$ has beneficial effects on the nerves, and therefore may help to prevent a number of neurological disorders as well as the numbness and tingling often associated with diabetes. It may also play a part in treating depression.

ADDITIONAL BENEFITS: Research shows that low levels of vitamin B$_{12}$ are common in people with Alzheimer's disease. Whether the deficiency is a contributing factor to the disease or simply a result of it is unknown. The nutrient does, however, keep the immune system healthy. Some studies suggest that it lengthens the period of time between infection

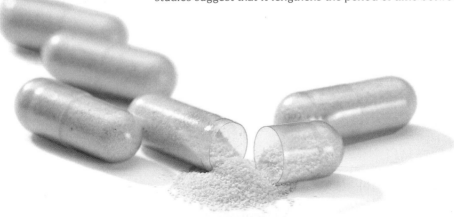

with the HIV virus and the development of AIDS. Other research indicates that adequate B_{12} intake improves immune responses in older people. With its beneficial effect on nerves, vitamin B_{12} may ease tinnitus (ringing in the ears). As a component of myelin it is valuable in treating multiple sclerosis, a disease that involves the destruction of this nerve covering.

How much you need

The recommended amount for vitamin B_{12} is 1.5 mcg a day for adults. Supplements of vitamin B_{12} may be important for older people and vegans (who eat no meat or dairy products).

IF YOU GET TOO LITTLE: Symptoms of a vitamin B_{12} deficiency include fatigue, depression, numbness and tingling in the extremities caused by nerve damage, muscle weakness, confusion and memory loss. Dementia and pernicious anaemia can develop; both are reversible if caught early.

The level of B_{12} in the blood decreases with age. People with ulcers, Crohn's disease or other gastrointestinal disorders are at risk, as are those taking prescription medication for epilepsy (seizures), chronic indigestion or gout. Excessive alcohol also hinders absorption of vitamin B_{12}.

IF YOU GET TOO MUCH: Excess vitamin B_{12} is readily excreted in urine, and there are no known adverse effects from a high intake of it.

How to take it

DOSAGE: A general dose of 1000 mcg of vitamin B_{12} a day may be useful for heart disease prevention, pernicious anaemia, numbness and tingling, tinnitus and multiple sclerosis. If you are deficient in B_{12}, higher doses may be needed. Or if you do not produce enough intrinsic factor, B_{12} injections or a prescription nasal spray may be necessary; ask your doctor for further information and guidance.

GUIDELINES FOR USE: Take vitamin B_{12} once a day, preferably in the morning, along with 400 mcg of folic acid. Most multivitamins contain at least the recommended amount of vitamin B_{12} and folic acid; B-complex supplements have higher amounts. For larger therapeutic amounts look for a supplement with just vitamin B_{12} or B_{12} with folic acid. Using a sublingual (under-the-tongue) form enhances absorption.

Other sources

Animal foods are the primary source of B_{12}. These include offal, brewer's yeast, oysters, sardines and other fish, eggs, meat and cheese. Many breakfast cereals are fortified with this vitamin as well.

Boost your vitamin B_{12} intake with cheese.

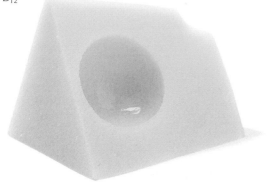

Vitamin C

Vitamin C is probably better known and more widely used than any other nutritional supplement, but even people who are particularly familiar with the uses of this versatile nutrient may be surprised to discover the extent of the health benefits it can provide.

Common uses

- *Enhances immunity.*
- *Minimises cold symptoms; shortens duration of illness.*
- *Speeds wound healing.*
- *Promotes healthy gums.*
- *Treats asthma.*
- *Helps to prevent cataracts.*
- *Protects against some forms of cancer and heart disease.*

Forms

- Capsule
- Liquid
- Powder
- Tablet

What it is

As early as 1742 lemon juice was known to prevent scurvy, a debilitating disease that often plagued long-distance sailors, but not until 1928 was the healthful component in lemon juice identified as vitamin C. Its anti-scurvy, or antiscorbutic, effect is the root of this vitamin's scientific name: ascorbic acid. Today, interest in vitamin C is based less on its ability to cure scurvy than on its potential to protect cells. As the body's primary water-soluble antioxidant, vitamin C helps to fight damage caused by unstable oxygen molecules called free radicals – especially in those areas that are mostly water, such as the interiors of cells.

What it does

Vitamin C is active throughout the body. It helps to strengthen the capillaries (the tiniest blood vessels) and cell walls and is crucial for the formation of collagen (a protein found in connective tissue). In these ways vitamin C prevents bruising, promotes healing and keeps ligaments (which connect muscle to bone), tendons (which connect bone to bone) and gums strong and healthy. It also aids the production of haemoglobin in red blood cells and helps the body to absorb iron from foods.

PREVENTION: As an antioxidant, vitamin C offers protection against cancer and heart disease; several studies have shown that low levels of this vitamin are linked to heart attacks. In addition, vitamin C may actually lengthen life. In one study, men who consumed more than 300 mg of vitamin C a day (from food and supplements) lived longer than men who consumed less than 50 mg a day.

Another study found that, over the long term, vitamin C supplements protect against cataracts, a clouding of the lens of the eye that interferes with vision. Women who took vitamin C for ten years or more had a 77% lower rate of early 'lens opacities', the first stage of cataracts, than women who did not take supplements.

ADDITIONAL BENEFITS: Does vitamin C prevent colds? Probably not, but it can help to lessen their symptoms and may shorten their duration. In a 1995 analysis of studies exploring the connection between vitamin C

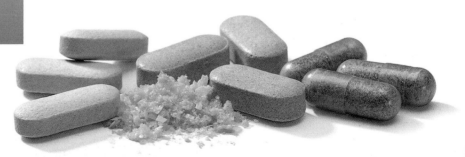

and colds, the researchers concluded that taking 1000 to 6000 mg a day at the onset of cold symptoms reduces the cold's duration by 21% – about one day. Other studies have shown that vitamin C helps elderly patients to fight severe respiratory infections. Vitamin C also appears to be a natural antihistamine. High doses of the vitamin can block the effect of inflammatory substances produced by the body in response to pollen, pet hair or other allergens.

The vitamin is an effective asthma remedy as well. Numerous studies have found that vitamin C supplements helped to prevent or improve asthmatic symptoms. For people with type 1 diabetes, which interferes with the transport of vitamin C into cells, supplementing with 1000 to 3000 mg a day may prevent complications of the disease, such as eye problems and high cholesterol levels.

How much you need

The recommended target for vitamin C for men and women is 40 mg a day (80 mg for smokers). However, even conservative nutritionists think an optimal intake is at least 200 mg a day, and they recommend higher doses for the treatment of specific diseases.

⊖ **IF YOU GET TOO LITTLE:** You would have to consume less than 10 mg of vitamin C a day to get scurvy, but receiving less than 50 mg a day has been linked with a higher risk of heart attack, cataracts and a shorter life.

⊕ **IF YOU GET TOO MUCH:** Large doses of vitamin C – more than 1000 mg a day – can cause loose stools, diarrhoea, flatulence and bloating; all can be corrected by reducing your daily dose. At this level the vitamin may interfere with the absorption of copper and selenium, so make sure you consume enough of these minerals in food or supplements. Continued high doses of vitamin C may lead to the development of kidney stones in susceptible individuals.

How to take it

▨ **DOSAGE:** *For general health*: 200 mg of vitamin C a day through foods and supplements. *For the treatment of various diseases*: Depending on the condition, 1000 mg a day may be appropriate.

◉ **GUIDELINES FOR USE:** Large amounts are most easily absorbed in 200 mg doses, taken with meals throughout the day. The vitamin works very well when combined with other antioxidants, such as vitamin E.

Other sources

Citrus fruits and juices, broccoli, dark-green leafy vegetables, red peppers, strawberries and kiwi fruits are all good sources of vitamin C.

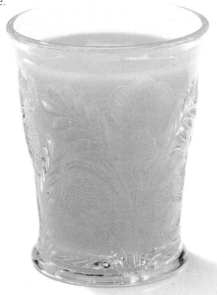

RECENT FINDINGS

Vitamin C may help to prevent reblockage (restenosis) of arteries after angioplasty (an alternative to bypass surgery). A study of 119 angioplasty patients found that restenosis occurred in just 24% of those who took 500 mg of vitamin C a day for four months, but in 43% of those who did not take the vitamin.

⸻

In addition to being an antioxidant, vitamin C helps the body to recycle other antioxidants. In one study, vitamin E concentrations were 18% higher in those who got more than 220 mg of vitamin C a day than in people who got 120 mg or less.

⸻

Vitamin C may help to prevent arthritis. A large study, involving 25,000 people, found that the risk of arthritis was significantly higher in those whose diet was low in vitamin C and fruit and vegetables.

DID YOU KNOW?

A 225 ml glass of freshly squeezed orange juice supplies 124 mg of vitamin C – well over half the daily target thought to be desirable for optimal health.

Vitamin D

Called the sunshine vitamin – because your body makes all it needs with enough sunlight – vitamin D is essential for healthy bones and may slow the progression of osteoporosis. It is also believed to strengthen the immune system and possibly prevent some cancers.

Common uses

- *Aids in the body's absorption of calcium.*
- *Promotes healthy bones.*
- *Strengthens teeth.*
- *May protect against some types of cancer.*

Forms

- Capsule
- Liquid
- Softgel
- Tablet

What it is

Technically a hormone, vitamin D is produced within the body when the skin is exposed to the ultraviolet B (UVB) rays in sunlight. Theoretically, spending a few minutes in the sun each day supplies all the vitamin D your body needs, but many people do not get enough sun to generate adequate vitamin D, especially in winter.

What is more, the body's ability to manufacture vitamin D declines with age, so vitamin D deficiencies are common in older people. But even young adults may not have sufficient vitamin D stores. One study of nearly 300 patients (of all ages) hospitalised for a variety of causes found that 57% of them did not have high enough levels of vitamin D. Of particular concern was the observation that a vitamin D deficiency was present in a third of the people who obtained the recommended amount of vitamin D through diet or supplements. This finding suggests that current recommendations for vitamin D may not be high enough.

What it does

The basic function of vitamin D is to regulate blood levels of calcium and phosphorus, helping to build strong bones and healthy teeth.

PREVENTION: Studies have shown that vitamin D is important in the prevention of osteoporosis, a disease that causes porous bones and thus an increased risk of fractures. Without sufficient vitamin D, the body cannot absorb calcium from food or supplements, no matter how much calcium you consume. When blood calcium levels are low, the body will move calcium from the bones to the blood to supply the muscles – especially those of the heart – and the nerves with the amount they need. Over time, this reallocation of calcium leads to a loss of bone mass.

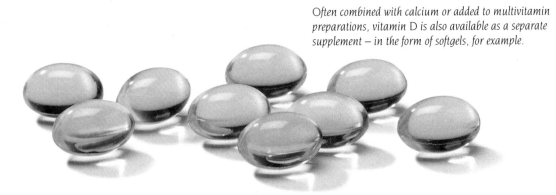

Often combined with calcium or added to multivitamin preparations, vitamin D is also available as a separate supplement – in the form of softgels, for example.

ADDITIONAL BENEFITS: Scientists are continuing to discover more about the functions of vitamin D in the body. Some studies suggest that it is important for a healthy immune system; others indicate that it may help to prevent prostate, colon or breast cancer. One study found that adequate vitamin D slowed the progression of osteoarthritis in the knees, although it did not prevent the disease from developing in the first place.

How much you need

A recommended daily target for vitamin D has not been set for adults because it is assumed that sufficient will be made through the action of sunlight on the skin. However, for people over 65, and for pregnant or breastfeeding women, the recommended target is 10 mcg a day.

IF YOU GET TOO LITTLE: A vitamin D deficiency can harm the bones, causing a bone-weakening disease in children (rickets) and increase the risk of osteoporosis in adults. A deficiency can also cause diarrhoea, insomnia, nervousness and muscle twitches. The likelihood of a child developing rickets today is remote, however, since children typically spend enough time in the sun to generate ample vitamin D.

IF YOU GET TOO MUCH: Although your body effectively rids itself of any extra vitamin D it makes from sunlight, too many supplements may create problems. Daily doses of 25 to 50 mcg over six months can cause constipation or diarrhoea, headache, loss of appetite, nausea and vomiting, heartbeat irregularities and extreme fatigue. Continued high doses can disrupt the balance of calcium and phosphate, weaken the bones and allow calcium to accumulate in soft tissues, such as muscles.

How to take it

DOSAGE: As little as 10 to 15 minutes of midday sunlight on your face, hands and arms two or three times a week can supply all the vitamin D you need. But if you are over 50, or you do not get outdoors much between the hours of 8am and 3pm or you always wear sunscreen, you might want to consider vitamin D supplements. Many practitioners recommend 10 to 15 mcg a day for people over 50, while 5 to 10 mcg a day is probably sufficient for younger adults.

GUIDELINES FOR USE: Supplements can be taken at any time of day, with or without food. Most daily multivitamins contain up to 10 mcg of vitamin D. It is also often found in calcium supplements.

Other sources

Many breakfast cereals are fortified with 1 to 2.5 mcg of vitamin D in each serving. Fatty fish, such as herring, salmon and tuna, are naturally rich in this vitamin.

RECENT FINDINGS

Vitamin D helps to protect post-menopausal women from hip fractures caused by osteoporosis. In a study involving 73,000 women, those taking 12.5 mcg of vitamin D from food plus supplements, had a 37 per cent lower risk of developing hip fractures than those consuming less than 3.5 mcg a day

Vitamin D may help to prevent colon cancer. In a study of 438 men, researchers found that those with colon cancer had lower blood levels of vitamin D than those who did not have the disease. Across the board, men with the highest vitamin D intake had the best chance of avoiding colon cancer. More study is needed to confirm this finding and to see if the risk is the same for women.

FACTS & TIPS

In northern latitudes the sun's rays are not strong enough to stimulate vitamin D production in winter. Everyone living in the UK is likely to be affected, but people living in Scotland are especially vulnerable. If you get enough exposure to the sun during the rest of the year, your body can store enough vitamin D to carry you through to spring. If you do not, consider taking a daily vitamin D supplement during the winter.

Vitamin E

A crucially important nutrient with antioxidant capability, vitamin E offers a multitude of benefits, including protection against heart disease, cancer and a range of other disorders. As it works at the body's cellular level, vitamin E may even slow down the ageing process.

Common uses

- Helps to protect against heart disease, certain cancers and various other chronic ailments.
- May delay or prevent cataracts.
- Enhances the immune system.
- Protects against toxins from cigarette smoke and other pollutants.
- Aids in skin healing.

Forms

- Capsule
- Cream
- Liquid
- Oil
- Softgel
- Tablet

CAUTION!

- People on prescription blood-thinning drugs (anticoagulants) or aspirin should consult their doctor before using vitamin E.

- Do not take vitamin E two days before or after surgery.

REMINDER: *If you have a medical condition, consult your doctor before taking supplements.*

What it is

Vitamin E is a generic term for a group of related compounds called tocopherols, which occur in four major forms: alpha, beta, gamma and delta-tocopherols. Alpha-tocopherol is the most common and most potent form of the vitamin. Vitamin E is fat-soluble, and so is stored for relatively long periods in the body, mainly in fat tissue and the liver. It is found in only a few foods, and many of these are high in fat, which makes it difficult to get the amount of vitamin E you require while on a low-fat diet. Supplements can therefore be very useful in obtaining optimal amounts of this nutrient.

What it does

One of vitamin E's basic functions is to protect cell membranes. It also helps the body to use selenium and vitamin K. But vitamin E's current reputation comes from its disease-fighting potential as an antioxidant – meaning that it assists in destroying or neutralising free radicals, the unstable oxygen molecules that cause damage to cells.

PREVENTION: By safeguarding cell membranes and acting as an antioxidant, vitamin E may play a role in preventing cancer. Some compelling research indicates that vitamin E can help to protect against cardiovascular disease, including heart attacks and strokes, by reducing the harmful effects of LDL ('bad') cholesterol and by preventing blood clots. In addition, vitamin E may offer protection because it works to reduce inflammatory processes that have been linked to heart disease. Findings from two large studies suggest that vitamin E may reduce the risk of heart disease by 25% to 50% – and it may prevent chest pain (angina) as well. Recent findings suggest that taking vitamin E with vitamin C may help to block some of the harmful effects of a fatty meal.

ADDITIONAL BENEFITS: Vitamin E protects cells from free-radical damage, which leads some clinicians to think that vitamin E may retard the ageing process. There is also evidence to suggest that it improves

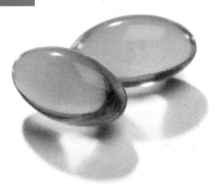
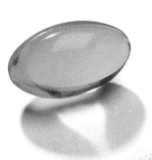

The vitamin E oil contained in softgels can be used to heal minor skin wounds.

immune function in the elderly, combats toxins from cigarette smoke and other pollutants, postpones the development of cataracts and slows the progression of Alzheimer's disease – and perhaps of Parkinson's disease.

Other research found that vitamin E can relieve the severe leg pain caused by a circulatory problem called intermittent claudication. It may alleviate premenstrual breast pain and tenderness as well. In addition, many people report that applying creams or oils containing vitamin E to skin wounds helps to promote healing.

How much you need

Although a recommended daily amount for vitamin E has not been set, recommended safe intakes are 4 mg a day for men and 3 mg a day for women. Safe intake levels may be enough to prevent deficiency, but higher doses are needed to provide the full antioxidant effect.

⊖ **IF YOU GET TOO LITTLE:** When the levels of vitamin E consumed are below the recommended safe intakes, neurological damage may occur and the life of red blood cells may be shortened. However, people who eat a balanced diet are unlikely to be at risk.

⊕ **IF YOU GET TOO MUCH:** No toxic effects from large doses of vitamin E have been discovered. Minor effects, such as headaches and diarrhoea, have rarely been reported. But large doses of vitamin E can interfere with the absorption of vitamin A.

How to take it

▢ **DOSAGE:** Many nutritionists recommend that, to benefit from the disease-fighting potential of vitamin E, you should take 250 to 500 mg daily in capsule or tablet form. (This total includes amounts obtained from a multivitamin.) Doses of up to 800 mg have been recommended for those at high risk of heart disease and certain cancers. It may be particularly effective when taken with vitamin C.

◉ **GUIDELINES FOR USE:** Try to take vitamin E supplements at the same time each day. Combining it with a meal decreases stomach irritation and increases the absorption of this fat-soluble vitamin. For topical use, break open a capsule and apply the oil directly to your skin, or use a commercial cream containing vitamin E as needed.

Other sources

Wheat germ is an outstanding dietary source of vitamin E: 2 tablespoons contain the equivalent of 40 mg. Beneficial amounts of vitamin E are also found in vegetable oils, nuts and seeds (such as almonds and sunflower seeds), green leafy vegetables and whole grains.

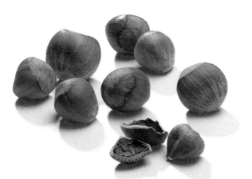

Hazelnuts are one of the foods that offer a good source of vitamin E.

Vitamin K

Doctors have long used vitamin K, which promotes blood clotting, to help to reduce blood loss after surgery and to prevent bleeding problems in newborn babies. This vitamin also aids in building strong bones and may be useful for combating the threat of osteoporosis.

Common uses

- *Reduces the risk of internal haemorrhaging.*
- *Protects against bleeding problems after surgery.*
- *Helps to build strong bones, and to ward off or treat osteoporosis.*

Forms

- Liquid
- Tablet

CAUTION!

- Supplemental vitamin K (more than is found in a multivitamin) should be taken only with your doctor's supervision.

REMINDER: If you have a medical condition, consult your doctor before taking supplements.

What it is

In the 1930s Danish researchers noticed that baby chickens fed a fat-free diet developed bleeding problems. They eventually solved the problem with an alfalfa-based compound that they named vitamin K, for *Koagulation*. Scientists now know that most of the body's vitamin K needs are met by the beneficial activity of bacteria in the intestines that produce this vitamin, and only about 20% comes from foods. Deficiencies are rare in healthy people, even though the body does not store vitamin K in high amounts. Synthetic supplements are available by prescription. Other names for vitamin K are phytonadione and menadiol.

What it does

This single nutrient sets in motion the entire blood-clotting process as soon as a wound occurs. Without it, we might bleed to death. Researchers have discovered that vitamin K plays a protective role in bone health as well.

PREVENTION: Doctors may recommend preventative doses of vitamin K if bleeding or haemorrhaging is a concern. Even when no deficiency exists, surgeons frequently order vitamin K before an operation to reduce the risk of postoperative bleeding. Under medical supervision it can also be prescribed for excessive menstrual bleeding. Though it is not yet a widely accepted treatment, vitamin K may provide benefits for those suffering from osteoporosis. Some studies show that it helps the body to make use of calcium and decreases the risk of fractures. Vitamin K may be especially important for bone health in older women. Not surprisingly, it is included among the ingredients in many bone-building formulas.

ADDITIONAL BENEFITS: Vitamin K may play a role in cancer prevention and help those undergoing radiation therapy. Recent findings also put vitamin K in the arsenal of heart-supporting nutrients: some evidence suggests it may halt the build-up of disease-causing plaque in arteries and reduce the blood level of LDL ('bad') cholesterol. But more research is needed to define the role of vitamin K in these and other disorders.

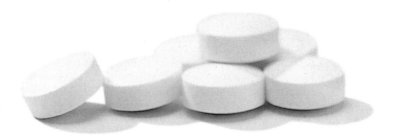

How much you need

Although a recommended daily amount for vitamin K has not been set, the recommended safe intake for adults is 1 mcg a day per 1 kilogram of body weight.

IF YOU GET TOO LITTLE: In healthy people, a vitamin K deficiency is rare because the body manufactures most of what it requires. In fact, deficiencies are found only in those with liver disease or intestinal illnesses that interfere with fat absorption. However, vitamin K levels can drop as a result of long-term use of antibiotics. One of the first signs of a deficiency is a tendency to bruise easily. Those at risk need careful medical monitoring because they could bleed to death in the event of a serious injury.

IF YOU GET TOO MUCH: It is hard to get too much vitamin K because it is not abundant in any one food (except leafy greens). Although even megadoses are not toxic, high doses can be dangerous if you are taking anticoagulants. Large doses also may cause flushing and sweating.

How to take it

DOSAGE: Multivitamins often contain between 25 and 60 mcg of vitamin K. Bone-building formulas provide around 300 mcg a day, the equivalent of adding a large leafy salad to your daily diet. Higher doses (such as those in prenatal multivitamins) may be prescribed under medical supervision for those with specific medical needs.

GUIDELINES FOR USE: When prescribed, vitamin K should be taken with meals to enhance absorption.

Other sources

Leafy green vegetables, including – per serving – kale (550 mcg) and Swiss chard (300 mcg), are richest in vitamin K. Broccoli, spring onions and brussels sprouts are also good sources. Other foods with some vitamin K are pistachio nuts, vegetable oils, meats and dairy products.

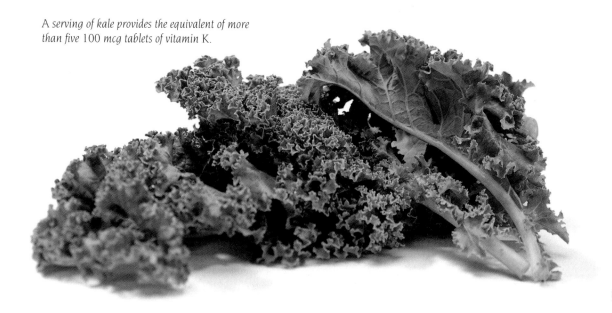

A serving of kale provides the equivalent of more than five 100 mcg tablets of vitamin K.

White willow bark

Used for thousands of years to treat fevers and headaches, white willow bark contains a chemical forerunner of today's most popular painkiller – aspirin. The herb is sometimes called 'herbal aspirin' but has few of that drug's side effects.

Salix alba

Common uses

- *Relieves acute and chronic pains, including back and neck pain, headaches and muscle aches.*
- *Reduces arthritis inflammation.*
- *May lower fevers.*

Forms

- Capsule
- Dried herb/tea
- Powder
- Tablet
- Tincture

CAUTION!

- Avoid white willow bark if you are allergic to aspirin. When subject to fever, children and teenagers should also avoid the herb.

- Pregnant or breastfeeding women should consult their doctors before taking white willow bark, because its safety has not been established in these situations.

REMINDER: If you have a medical condition, consult your doctor before taking supplements.

What it is

White willow bark comes from the stately white willow tree, which can grow up to 23 metres tall. In China its medicinal properties have been appreciated for centuries, but not until the 18th century was the herb recognised as a pain reliever and fever reducer in the West. European settlers brought the white willow tree to North America, where they discovered that local tribes were already using native willow species to alleviate pain and fight fevers.

In 1828 the plant's active ingredient, salicin, was isolated by German and French scientists. Ten years later, European chemists manufactured from it salicylic acid, a chemical cousin to aspirin. Aspirin, or acetyl-salicylic acid, was later created from a different salicin-containing herb called meadowsweet. By the end of the 19th century the Bayer Company had begun commercially producing aspirin, which was marketed as a new and safer pain reliever than wintergreen and black birch oil, the herbs commonly employed at that time for reducing pain.

All parts of the white willow contain salicin, but concentrations of this chemical are highest in the bark, which is collected in early spring from trees that are two to five years old. *Salix alba*, or white willow, is the most popular species for medicinal use, but other types of willow are also rich in salicin, including *Salix fragilis* (crack willow), *Salix purpurea* (purple willow) and *Salix daphnoides* (violet willow). These species are often sold simply as willow bark in health-food shops.

What it does

In the body, the salicin from white willow bark is metabolised to form salicylic acid, which reduces pain, fever and inflammation. Though the

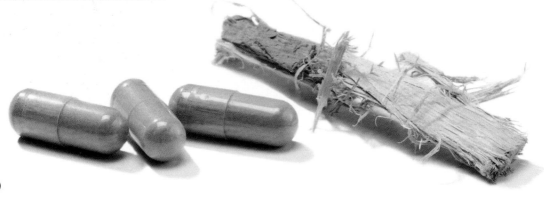

Bark from the white willow tree – dried, concentrated, and packaged into capsules or tablets – is the source of a potent natural pain reliever.

herb is slower acting than aspirin, its beneficial effects last longer, and it causes fewer adverse reactions. Most notably, it does not produce stomach bleeding – one of aspirin's most potentially serious side effects.

✴ **MAJOR BENEFITS:** White willow bark can be very effective for relieving headaches as well as acute muscle aches and pains. It can also alleviate all sorts of chronic pain, including back and neck pain. When recommended for arthritis, especially if there is pain in the back, knees, and hips, it can reduce swelling and inflammation and increase joint mobility. In addition it may help to ease the pain of menstrual cramps – the salicin interferes with the action of hormone-like chemicals called prostaglandins that can contribute to inflammation and cause pain.

✴ **ADDITIONAL BENEFITS:** White willow bark, like aspirin, may be useful for alleviating fevers.

How to take it

⊘ **DOSAGE:** Take one or two capsules or tablets three times a day, or as needed to relieve pain, calm a fever or reduce inflammation (follow the instructions on the packet). Look for preparations that are standardised to contain 15% salicin. This dosage provides between 60 and 120 mg a day of salicin. Standardised extracts can also be taken in tincture or powder form. White willow bark teas are likely to be less effective than standardised extracts because they supply only a small amount of pain-relieving salicin.

◎ **GUIDELINES FOR USE:** White willow bark is safe to use long term. It has a bitter, astringent taste, so the most convenient way to take it is probably in capsule or tablet form. Do not consume white willow bark with aspirin because it can amplify the side effects of aspirin.

As a precaution, do not give the herb to a child or teenager under 16 who has a cold, flu or chicken pox. Taking aspirin can put these young people at risk of a potentially fatal brain and liver condition called Reye's syndrome. Salicin, the therapeutic ingredient in white willow bark, is unlikely to cause this problem because it is metabolised differently from aspirin, but its similarities to the painkiller warrant a cautious approach. Paracetamol is a better choice than white willow bark or aspirin for children and teenagers.

Possible side effects

This herb rarely causes side effects at recommended doses. However, higher doses can lead to an upset stomach, nausea or tinnitus. If any of these occur, lower the dosage or stop taking the herb. Consult your doctor if side effects persist.

BUYING GUIDE

■ Buy white willow bark extract standardised to contain 15% salicin – the aspirin-like active ingredient in the herb.

■ White willow bark tea may be recommended as a pain reliever, but you should take only the standardised extracts, in capsule or tablet, powder or tincture form. Because the bark contains 1% or less salicin, you'd probably have to drink several litres of tea to get an effective dose.

■ If white willow bark does not help to alleviate pain, you can try other pain-relieving herbs, such as meadowsweet, feverfew, ginger, cat's claw, pau d'arco or turmeric.

RECENT FINDINGS

A recent study confirms earlier reports that white willow bark appears to be quite safe. Among 41 patients with long-standing arthritis who were treated for two months with white willow bark (as well as other herbs), only three people taking the herbs had mild adverse reactions, including headache and digestive upset – all of which also occurred in those who were given a placebo.

DID YOU KNOW?

Native Americans and early settlers believed in chewing willow twigs 'until your ears ring' to relieve headache pain. Ringing in the ears is now seen as a sign that you've taken too much of the herb or its drug counterpart, aspirin.

Wild yam

Dioscorea villosa

Common uses

- *Relieves menstrual cramps.*
- *May ease the pain of endometriosis.*
- *Reduces inflammation.*

Forms

- Capsule
- Cream
- Dried herb/tea
- Softgel
- Tablet
- Tincture

CAUTION!

- **Pregnant women should not use wild yam.**

REMINDER: If you have a medical condition, consult your doctor before taking supplements.

Misconceptions about the active ingredients in wild yam have led to exaggerated claims. The herb has been hailed as a natural alternative to hormone replacement therapy following the menopause. Wild yam has not been proved effective for this purpose, but it does have other benefits.

What it is

In some countries 'yam' describes a type of sweet potato with reddish flesh. This vegetable is not related, even distantly, to wild yam, a native plant of North and Central America that was first used medicinally by the Aztecs and Mayas for its pain-relieving qualities. Later, European settlers took advantage of the wild yam's therapeutic properties and utilised it for treating joint pain and colic. The root is the part of the plant that has medicinal value. Sold as a dried herb for use in tea, it is also available in several other forms.

What it does

In recent years wild yam has been extolled for its ability to mimic certain hormones – especially progesterone – and said to relieve menopausal or PMS symptoms. Most of these claims remain scientifically unproven, however. It is true that wild yam contains a substance called diosgenin that can be converted to progesterone in the laboratory, but the human body is unable to make this conversion.

Some holistic practitioners have reported that patients suffering from premenstrual syndrome (PMS) and menopausal symptoms experienced good results with wild yam cream, which is applied to the soft areas of

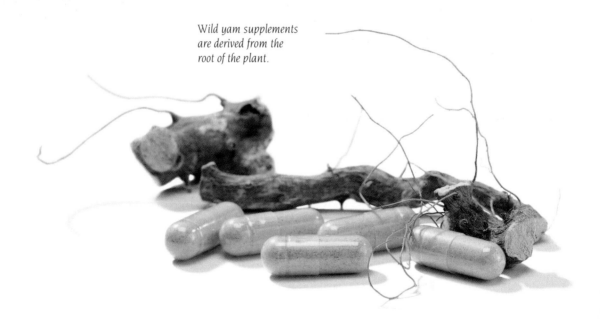

Wild yam supplements are derived from the root of the plant.

the body (abdomen and thighs). How the cream helps is unclear. Sometimes manufacturers of the creams add laboratory-synthesised progesterone, which could well account for some of the therapeutic effects. Despite positive reports from patients, the value of pure wild yam creams has yet to be scientifically proven.

When taken in any of the available forms, wild yam does have other medicinal effects. Some herbalists believe that crude forms of it may help to rectify hormonal imbalances associated with PMS and the menopause because it contains oestrogen-like substances. In addition, wild yam acts as a muscle relaxant, antispasmodic and anti-inflammatory, which may explain why it alleviates menstrual complaints in some women.

✴ **MAJOR BENEFITS:** Wild yam contains substances called alkaloids, which are muscle relaxants that especially target muscles in the abdomen and pelvis. This action suggests that wild yam may be of value in treating digestive disorders such as Crohn's disease and irritable bowel syndrome. It can also ease menstrual cramps and the pain associated with endometriosis, a disorder of the uterine lining.

Some women find that wild yam combined with another herb, such as chasteberry, is particularly effective in relieving the symptoms of PMS; this is the result of both normalisation of hormone balance and anti-inflammatory action.

✴ **ADDITIONAL BENEFITS:** Other active ingredients found in wild yam, known as steroidal saponins, play a role in alleviating muscle strains, chronic muscle pain and arthritis.

How to take it

✐ **DOSAGE:** In order to receive the therapeutic benefits of wild yam, take a ½ teaspoon of tincture three or four times a day, or 500 mg of wild yam in capsule, tablet or softgel form twice a day. If you prefer, drink a cup of wild yam tea three times a day.

◉ **GUIDELINES FOR USE:** Take wild yam supplements or tincture with food to minimise the risk of stomach upsets. To make wild yam tea, pour a cup of very hot water over 1 or 2 teaspoons of the dried herb and let it steep for 15 minutes. You can add other soothing herbs to the tea – valerian or peppermint, for example – when using it for digestive disorders.

Possible side effects

In extremely large amounts wild yam supplements and tinctures can cause nausea and diarrhoea.

DID YOU KNOW?
The first contraceptive pill to be produced was derived from diosgenin, the hormone-like compound found in wild yam.

Zinc

Every cell in the body needs zinc, but many of us do not get enough of this vital mineral. Zinc is contained in enzymes – chemicals that do everything from digesting food to healing wounds. It is a crucial component of the immune system, helping to fight infections, including the common cold.

Common uses

- *Helps to prevent colds, flu and other infections.*
- *Helps to treat a wide range of chronic ailments, from rheumatoid arthritis and underactive thyroid to chronic fatigue and osteoporosis.*
- *Alleviates skin problems and digestive complaints.*
- *May improve fertility, build healthy hair and diminish tinnitus.*

Forms

- Capsule
- Liquid
- Lozenge
- Tablet

CAUTION!

■ Do not take too much zinc. More than 30 mg daily can, in the long term, interfere with copper absorption, leading to anaemia. Daily doses of more than 100 mg of zinc can also impair immunity.

REMINDER: If you have a medical condition, consult your doctor before taking supplements.

What it is

Zinc is concentrated in the muscles, bones, skin, kidneys, liver, pancreas, eyes and, in men, the prostate. It is plentiful in high-protein foods such as meat and fish. The body does not produce or store zinc, so it depends on external sources for a continuous supply.

What it does

Zinc is critical for hundreds of processes that take place in the body, from cell growth to sexual maturation and immunity – even for taste and smell. Consequently, everyone who takes a daily multivitamin and mineral supplement should make sure that it contains zinc.

✪ **MAJOR BENEFITS:** Necessary for the proper functioning of the immune system, zinc helps to protect the body against colds, flu, conjunctivitis and other infections. In an American study of 100 people in the initial stages of a cold, those who sucked zinc lozenges every couple of hours recovered from their illness about three days earlier than those who sucked placebo lozenges. Zinc lozenges may also speed the healing of mouth ulcers and sore throats. Taken as a dietary supplement, zinc may support the body's natural defence and repair systems in treating more serious illnesses, such as rheumatoid arthritis, lupus, chronic fatigue syndrome and possibly multiple sclerosis, as well as other conditions, such as AIDS, which are associated with an impaired immune system.

✪ **ADDITIONAL BENEFITS:** Zinc exerts beneficial effects on the production of various hormones, including the sex and thyroid hormones. It could be helpful for enhancing the fertility of both men and women, and is also important for the health of the prostate gland. In addition, it may be effective for people with underactive thyroids and, because it improves insulin levels, it may help those with diabetes. The fact that zinc is involved in so many systems of the body means that it has other

When taken as dietary supplements, zinc tablets (below left) should always include copper; zinc lozenges (below right), which often contain vitamin C, ward off the symptoms of colds and flu.

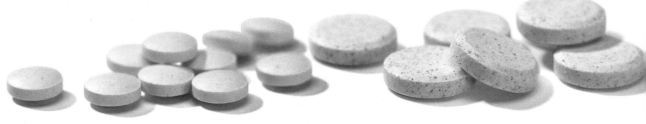

functions too. It stimulates the healing of wounds and skin irritations, which makes it a useful treatment for acne, burns, eczema, psoriasis and rosacea, and it promotes the health of the hair and scalp. Zinc has also been shown to slow vision loss in people with macular degeneration, a common cause of blindness in those aged over 50. In a recent Japanese study, tinnitus (ringing in the ears) improved with zinc supplementation. Zinc may also be useful for alleviating osteoporosis, haemorrhoids, inflammatory bowel disease and ulcers.

How much you need

The current recommended target for zinc is 7 mg for women and 9.5 mg for men daily. Higher doses are usually reserved for specific complaints.

⊟ **IF YOU GET TOO LITTLE:** Severe zinc deficiency is rare in the UK, but a mild zinc deficiency can lead to poor wound healing, more frequent colds and flu, a depressed sense of taste and smell, and skin problems such as acne, eczema and psoriasis. It can result in impaired blood sugar tolerance (and an increased diabetes risk) and a low sperm count.

⊕ **IF YOU GET TOO MUCH:** Long-term use of more than 100 mg a day has been shown to impair immunity and lower the level of HDL ('good') cholesterol. One study reported a connection between excessive zinc and Alzheimer's disease, though evidence is scant. Larger doses (more than 200 mg a day) can cause nausea, vomiting and diarrhoea.

How to take it

⊘ **DOSAGE:** The recommended target is 15 mg once a day. Taking high levels of zinc for longer than a month may interfere with copper absorption, so dietary supplements should include 2 mg of copper for every 30 mg of zinc. *For colds and flu*: Use zinc lozenges every 2 to 4 hours for a week; do not exceed 150 mg a day.

◉ **GUIDELINES FOR USE:** Take zinc an hour before or two hours after a meal; if it causes stomach upset, have it with a low-fibre food. If you are taking iron supplements for a specific condition, do not take them at the same time as zinc. Take zinc at least two hours after taking antibiotics.

Other sources

When looking for foods rich in zinc, think protein. It is abundant in beef, pork, liver, poultry (especially dark meat), eggs and seafood (especially oysters). Cheese, beans, nuts and wheat germ are other good sources, but the zinc in these foods is less easily absorbed than the zinc in meat.

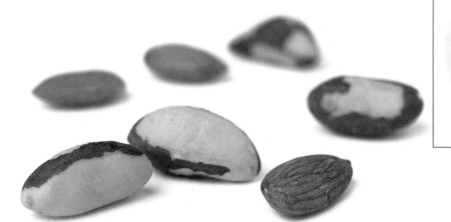

Drug interactions

Vitamins, minerals and other supplements are not safe to use in all circumstances. Some may interact adversely with prescription or over-the-counter (OTC) drugs, intensifying the action of the medications or even producing dangerous side effects.

This section lists most of the popular classes of drug and highlights reactions that may occur when specific supplements interact with them. Few studies have been done to determine the risks involved in taking supplements and medications together. Further research is needed, and caution is always advisable when combining any supplements with drugs.

To find out more about specific supplements listed here, refer to the individual entries in the A-Z of supplements on pages 22–175 of this book.

CHECKING FOR POSSIBLE INTERACTIONS

If you are taking a drug for a particular condition, scan the general categories listed alphabetically on the right to see if your drug presents a potential problem if used together with a particular supplement.

The most popular members of each drug class are listed by generic name, but not every drug in the group is included. (If you have any questions, consult your doctor or pharmacist.) Remember that all drugs within a category are likely to have similar interactions. Even if you don't see the name of your particular medication listed, the interaction may nevertheless apply to all the drugs in that class.

CONSULTING YOUR DOCTOR

Unless your doctor recommends it, avoid taking drugs and supplements with similar effects. For example, if you are using a herb such as kava or valerian to treat insomnia, it may induce excessive sleepiness when combined with a conventional sleeping aid or with any drug that can cause drowsiness – a narcotic pain reliever, an OTC antihistamine, or even alcohol.

Similarly, if you are already taking a prescription antidepressant, a nutritional supplement that affects brain chemicals and enhances mood, such as 5-HTP, is best tried only under the supervision of a doctor.

If you are taking any type of prescription drug you should not stop taking it without your doctor's advice or consent. If you have a medical or psychiatric condition, or are taking any prescription or OTC medication, always consult your doctor or pharmacist before trying any herb or supplement.

■ **BETAINE HCI** increases levels of digestive acids in the stomach. People taking aspirin or other anti-inflammatory medicines (NSAIDs) must avoid this supplement, because the combination increases the risk of stomach bleeding.

■ **GYMNEMA SYLVESTRE** may alter required dosages for insulin or oral diabetes drugs; consult your doctor before taking this herb with any medication for diabetes.

■ **PSYLLIUM** should not be used within 2 hours of taking any drug as it may delay absorption of the drug.

■ **ST JOHN'S WORT** interacts with several medicines, and can increase or decrease their effectiveness. Consult your doctor before taking this herb with any other medi-cation or supplement.

■ **VALERIAN** may cause excessive drowsiness in those people who are also using sedatives or drugs with sedative effects.

ACNE DRUGS
Isotretinoin and other acne drugs
Supplement interactions:
■ **VITAMIN A** if taken together with acne drugs, may cause high blood levels of vitamin A, increasing the chance of side effects.

ANTACIDS – ALL
Supplement interactions:
■ **FOLIC ACID** absorption is decreased by antacids; take folic acid supplements either 2 hours before or 2 hours after an antacid.

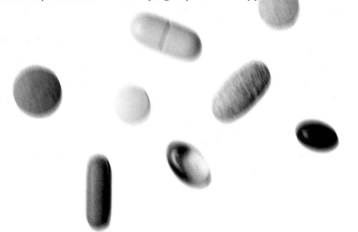

ANTIBIOTICS
All oral antibiotics
Supplement interactions:

■ **IRON** may make the antibiotic less effective; take iron supplements either 2 hours before or 2 hours after the drug.

Doxycycline, Minocycline and Tetracycline
Supplement interactions:

■ **BROMELAIN** may enhance absorption of amoxicillin, which is not necessarily a negative effect.

■ **CALCIUM** may decrease absorption of the drug; avoid taking calcium within 1 to 3 hours of taking any of these antibiotics.

■ **IRON** may make the antibiotic less effective; take iron supplements either 2 hours before or 2 hours after the drug.

■ **MAGNESIUM** may make the antibiotic less effective; take magnesium supplements 1 to 3 hours before or after the drug.

■ **PSYLLIUM** may make the antibiotic less effective; consult your doctor.

■ **VITAMIN C** may enhance absorption of tetracycline, which is not necessarily a negative effect.

■ **ZINC** may make the antibiotic less effective; take zinc supplements at least 2 hours after the drug.

ANTICOAGULANTS
Enoxaparin, Warfarin and other anti-coagulants (*blood thinners*)
Supplement interactions:

■ **BROMELAIN** use with caution; intensifies the blood-thinning effect of the medication; may lead to excessive bleeding.

■ **FEVERFEW** use with caution; intensifies the blood-thinning effect of the medication; may lead to excessive bleeding.

■ **FISH OILS** use with caution; intensifies the blood-thinning effect of the medication; may eventually lead to internal or excessive bleeding.

■ **GARLIC** may intensify the blood-thinning effect of the medication; consult your doctor before taking the two together.

■ **MEDICINAL MUSHROOMS** reishi mushrooms may intensify the blood-thinning effect of the medication; consult your doctor.

■ **PAU D'ARCO** use with caution; intensifies the blood-thinning effect of the medication; may lead to excessive bleeding.

■ **ST JOHN'S WORT** may enhance liver function, and could also reduce the effectiveness of anticoagulants; consult your doctor before taking this herb.

■ **VITAMIN E** may intensify the blood-thinning effect of the medication; consult your doctor before taking together.

■ **VITAMIN K** may counteract the effects of the medication.

ANTIDEPRESSANTS
Prozac and other antidepressants
Supplement interactions:

■ **5-HTP** avoid taking within four weeks of using a monoamine-oxidase (MAO) inhibitor; may cause anxiety, confusion and other potentially serious side effects; consult your doctor before combining with conventional anti-depressants.

■ **GINSENG (PANAX)** consult your doctor if you are taking an MAO inhibitor.

■ **ST JOHN'S WORT** taking this herb with conventional antidepressants may lead to adverse reactions; consult your doctor.

ANTIHISTAMINES
Supplement interactions:

■ **5-HTP, VALERIAN** any of these may cause excessive drowsiness when taken with sedative antihistamines.

CHOLESTEROL DRUGS
Atorvastatin, Lovastatin, Simvastatin and other 'statin' drugs
Supplement interactions:

■ **SOLUBLE FIBRE** may reduce absorption of these drugs; avoid excessive consumption.

COLD REMEDIES
OTC Prescription remedies containing ephedrine or pseudephedrine
Supplement interactions:

■ **5-HTP** may cause anxiety, confusion or other serious side effects if taken with these cold remedies; use with caution.

DIABETES DRUGS
Insulin and oral diabetes drugs
Supplement interactions:

■ **ALPHA-LIPOIC ACID** long-term use of supplements may require a change in dosage of insulin or diabetes medication.

■ **CAT'S CLAW** do not take with glipizide; adverse effects have been reported.

■ **CHROMIUM** may alter required dosages of insulin or other drugs; consult your doctor.

■ **DANDELION** use with caution; may intensify the blood-sugar-lowering effect of glipizide.

■ **GINSENG (PANAX)** long-term use of supplements may require a change in the dosage of insulin or other diabetes medications; check with your doctor.

■ **GINSENG (SIBERIAN)** use with caution; may intensify the blood-sugar-lowering effect of glipizide.

■ **GYMNEMA SYLVESTRE** may require a change in the dosage of insulin or other diabetes medications; consult your doctor.

DIURETICS
Amiloride, Spironolactone and Triamterene (*potassium-sparing diuretics*)
Supplement interactions:

■ **PHOSPHORUS** when used with phosphates containing potassium, phosphorus may increase the risk of hyperkalaemia (too much potassium in the blood), possibly leading to serious side effects; consult your doctor before taking together.

■ **POTASSIUM** do not take with diuretics; may increase the risk of hyperkalaemia (too much potassium in the blood), possibly leading to serious side effects.

Bumetanide, Ethacrynic acid, Furosemide and Torsemide (*loop diuretics*)
Supplement interactions:

■ **DANDELION** may boost the diuretic effects of these drugs if taken in high doses.

■ **GINSENG (PANAX)** if you are taking furosemide, may intensify the blood-pressure-lowering effects of the drug.

- **GLUCOSAMINE** higher doses of the diuretic may be necessary.

Chlorothiazide, Hydrochlorothiazide and Indapamide (*thiazide diuretics*)

Supplement interactions:

- **CALCIUM** may cause build-up of excessive, possibly toxic, calcium levels in the body, leading to kidney failure, if taken with a thiazide diuretic; consult your doctor.
- **DANDELION** may boost the diuretic effects of these drugs if taken in high doses.
- **GLUCOSAMINE** higher doses of the drug may be necessary.
- **LIQUORICE** may lead to dangerously low levels of potassium in the body; deglycyrrhised liquorice (DGL) should be taken instead.
- **POTASSIUM** if taking together with thiazide diuretic, do not suddenly discontinue the use of the diuretic; it may cause hyperkalaemia (too much potassium in the blood), possibly resulting in serious side effects.
- **VITAMIN D** may cause build-up of excessive – possibly toxic – levels of calcium in the body, resulting in kidney failure; consult your doctor.

HEART/BLOOD PRESSURE DRUGS

All antihypertensives

Supplement interactions:

- **BLACK COHOSH** may intensify the drug's effect of lowering blood pressure.
- **CALCIUM SUPPLEMENTS** may reduce blood pressure; consult your doctor.

- **GARLIC** may increase the potency of blood pressure medication; consult your doctor.
- **GINSENG (PANAX OR SIBERIAN)** consult your doctor if you are taking blood pressure medications.
- **HAWTHORN** may intensify the drug's effect of lowering blood pressure. A lower dose of the medication may be advisable; consult your doctor.
- **VITAMIN D** may reduce blood pressure; consult your doctor.

Amlodipine, Diltiazem, Verapamil and other calcium channel blockers

Supplement interactions:

- **FLAVONOIDS** when using a calcium channel blocker do not take a citrus bioflavonoid preparation containing naringin (a flavonoid that is present in grapefruit but not in oranges).

Benazepril, Enalapril, Fosinopril and other ACE inhibitors

Supplement interactions:

- **PHOSPHORUS** do not take together; when used with phosphates containing potassium, may increase the risk of hyperkalaemia (too much potassium in the blood) and lead to serious side effects.
- **POTASSIUM** do not take together; may increase the risk of hyperkalaemia (too much potassium in the blood) and lead to serious side effects.

Digitoxin and Digoxin (*digitalis drugs, cardiac glycosides*)

Supplement interactions:

- **GINSENG (SIBERIAN)** increases medication levels needed; consult your doctor before using them together.
- **HAWTHORN** may intensify the drug's effect of lowering blood pressure, so a lower dose of the medication may be advisable; consult your doctor.
- **PHOSPHORUS** using digitalis with phosphates containing potassium may increase the risk of hyperkalaemia (too much potassium in the blood), possibly leading to serious side effects; consult your doctor.
- **POTASSIUM** when taken together, may increase the risk of hyperkalaemia (too much potassium in the blood), possibly leading to serious side effects; consult your doctor before taking together.

Amyl nitrite, Isosorbide mononitrate or dinitrate and Nitroglycerin (*Nitrates*)

Supplement interactions:

- **NAC (N-ACETYLCYSTEINE)** do not take with nitrates; this may cause severe headaches.

MUSCLE RELAXANTS

Carisoprodol, Cyclobenzaprine and other muscle relaxants

Supplement interactions:

- **5-HTP, VALERIAN** either of these may cause excessive drowsiness when taken with muscle relaxants.

NARCOTIC PAIN RELIEVERS

Codeine, Hydrocodone/ Acetaminophen and other narcotic analgesics

Supplement interactions:

- **5-HTP, VALERIAN** either of these may cause excessive drowsiness when taken with narcotic pain relievers.

NEUROLOGY DRUGS

Methylphenidate (*Ritalin*) and other nervous system stimulants

Supplement interactions:

- **FLAVONOIDS** use with caution when taking a citrus bioflavonoid preparation containing naringin (a flavonoid present in grapefruit but not in oranges) with methylphenidate.
- **GINSENG (PANAX)** increases the risk of overstimulation of the nervous system and stomach upset.

NONSTEROIDAL ANTI-INFLAMMATORY DRUGS (NSAIDs)

Etodolac, Ibuprofen, Ketoprofen, Naproxen and other NSAIDs

Supplement interactions:

- **BETAINE HCl** do not take together; increases the risk of potentially serious stomach bleeding.
- **PHOSPHORUS** when used with phosphates containing potassium, may increase the risk of hyperkalaemia (too much potassium in the blood), possibly leading to serious side effects; consult your doctor before taking with NSAIDs.
- **POTASSIUM** when taken together, may increase the risk of hyperkalaemia (too much potassium in the blood), possibly leading to serious side effects; consult your doctor.

Aspirin

Supplement interactions:

■ **BETAINE HCl** do not take together; increases the risk of potentially serious stomach bleeding.

■ **FEVERFEW** intensifies the blood-thinning effect of long-term aspirin use; may lead to excessive bleeding.

■ **FISH OILS** intensify the blood-thinning effect of long-term aspirin use; may lead to internal or excessive bleeding.

■ **GARLIC** may increase the blood-thinning effect of long-term aspirin use; consult your doctor.

■ **GINKGO BILOBA** intensifies the blood-thinning effect of long-term aspirin use; may lead to excessive bleeding.

■ **MEDICINAL MUSHROOMS** reishi mushrooms may intensify the blood-thinning effect of long-term aspirin use; consult your doctor.

■ **VITAMIN E** intensifies the blood-thinning effect caused by long-term aspirin use, and may lead to excessive bleeding.

■ **VITAMIN K** may counteract the blood-thinning effect of long-term aspirin use.

OBSTETRIC AND GYNAECOLOGICAL DRUGS

Conjugated oestrogens, Oestrogen-progestogen products and other female hormones

Supplement interactions:

■ **BLACK COHOSH** may interact adversely when taken together; consult your doctor.

■ **CAT'S CLAW** use with caution; may affect levels of female sex hormones.

■ **FLAVONOIDS** use with caution when taking a citrus bioflavonoid preparation containing naringin (a flavonoid which is present in grapefruit but not in oranges) together with oestrogens.

■ **ST JOHN'S WORT** may enhance liver function, resulting in decreased levels of oestrogen in the blood; consult your doctor before taking this herb.

Oral contraceptives (*combination oestrogen-progestogen products*)

Supplement interactions:

■ **BLACK COHOSH** may interact adversely; consult your doctor.

■ **CAT'S CLAW** use with caution; may affect levels of female sex hormones.

■ **ST JOHN'S WORT** may enhance liver function, resulting in decreased levels of oestrogen in the blood; consult your doctor before taking this herb.

PARKINSON'S DISEASE DRUGS

Levodopa

Supplement interactions:

■ **5-HTP** may cause anxiety, confusion and other serious side effects when taken together; consult your doctor.

■ **VITAMIN B$_6$** may prevent the medication from working properly.

PSYCHIATRIC DRUGS

Antipsychotics

Supplement interactions:

■ **GINSENG (PANAX)** consult your doctor if you are taking antipsychotics.

Buspirone (*anti-anxiety*)

Supplement interactions:

■ **5-HTP** may cause anxiety, confusion and other serious side effects when taken together; consult your doctor.

Lithium (*antimanic agent*)

Supplement interactions:

■ **5-HTP** may cause anxiety, confusion and other serious side effects when taken together; consult your doctor.

SEDATIVES AND TRANQUILLISERS

Sleeping aids and other sedatives

Supplement interactions:

■ **BLACK COHOSH, 5-HTP, VALERIAN** any of these may cause excessive drowsiness when taken with sedatives.

SEIZURE/EPILEPSY DRUGS

Carbamazepine, Gabapentin, Phenytoin and other anticonvulsants

Supplement interactions:

■ **FOLIC ACID** has been shown to interfere with some anticonvulsants when consumed in amounts exceeding a total daily dose of 1 mg; let your doctor know if you are taking folic acid and never exceed recommended dosages.

STEROIDS

Beclomethasone, Methylprednisolone, Prednisone and other oral corticosteroids

Supplement interactions:

■ **BETAINE HCl** do not take together.

■ **GINSENG (PANAX)** use with caution; may interact when taken together.

THYROID DRUGS

Methimazol and Propylthiouracil

Supplement interactions:

■ **IODINE** may decrease effectiveness of these and other antithyroid agents.

■ **KELP** taking high doses could provide too much iodine and interfere with the actions of these medications.

TRANSPLANT DRUGS

Cyclosporine and other immunosuppressants

Supplement interactions:

■ **FLAVONOIDS** do not take a citrus bioflavonoid preparation containing naringin (a flavonoid present in grapefruit but not in oranges) when using an immunosuppressant.

■ **ST JOHN'S WORT** may enhance liver function, and could reduce levels of immunosuppressive drugs; consult your doctor before taking this herb.

Useful addresses

The following organisations can provide information about nutritional and herbal therapies and practitioners.

BRITISH NUTRITION FOUNDATION
High Holborn House
52-54 High Holborn
London WC1V 6RQ
020 7404 6504
www.nutrition.org.uk
Provides fact sheets on various aspects of nutrition, but does not give nutritional advice to individuals.

BRITISH SOCIETY FOR ECOLOGICAL MEDICINE
PO Box 7
Knighton LD7 1WT
001547 550378
www.bsaenm.org
Society of doctors who emphasise the importance of nutritional therapy.

COMPLEMENTARY MEDICAL ASSOCIATION
67 Eagle Heights
The Falcons
Bramlands Close
London SW11 2LJ
0845 129 8434
www.the-cma.org.uk
Runs a free referral scheme for registered practitioners. Send two loose first-class stamps for details of qualified and insured practitioners in your area.

GENERAL COUNCIL AND REGISTER OF NATUROPATHS
Goswell House Clinic
2 Goswell Road
Street, Somerset BA16 0JG
0870 7456 984
www.naturopathy.org.uk
Provides a register of naturopaths, downloadable from the web site or by post from the secretary.

INSTITUTE FOR COMPLEMENTARY MEDICINE
PO Box 194,
London SE16 7QZ
020 7237 5165
www.i-c-m.org.uk
Provides information and has a searchable online database of accredited practitioners in a variety of disciplines.

INSTITUTE FOR OPTIMUM NUTRITION
Avalon House
72 Mortlake Road
Richmond, Surrey TW9 2JY
0870 979 1122
www.ion.ac.uk
Educational trust offering information service, courses and membership scheme.

INTERNATIONAL REGISTER OF CONSULTANT HERBALISTS AND HOMEOPATHS
32 King Edward Road
Swansea SA1 4LL
01792 655886
www.irch.org
Can provide a list of qualified practitioners.

NATIONAL INSTITUTE FOR MEDICAL HERBALISTS
Elm House,
54 Mary Arches Street
Exeter EX4 3BA
01392 426022
www.nimh.org.uk
Can provide a list of qualified practitioners.

NUTRITION SOCIETY
10 Cambridge Court
210 Shepherd's Bush Road
London W6 7NJ
020 7602 0228
www.nutritionsociety.org
Academic society which publishes scientific journals including the British Journal of Nutrition, which is also available on its web site.

The organisations listed below can give information, advice and support in relation to specific ailments.

ALLERGY UK
3 White Oak Square
London Road
Swanley, Kent BR8 7AG
01322 619 898
www.allergyuk.org
Runs a helpline offering support, details of your nearest allergy clinic, self-help and fact sheets.

ALZHEIMER'S SOCIETY
Gordon House
10 Greencoat Place
London SW1P 1PH
020 7306 0606
www.alzheimers.org.uk
Book ordering and library service, leaflets, information and advice.

ARTHRITIC ASSOCIATION
One Upperton Gardens
Eastbourne BN21 2AA
01323 416550
freefone: 0800 652 3188
www.arthriticassociation.org.uk
Offers membership and support, and gives advice on a home treatment plan using natural methods.

BRITISH ASSOCIATION OF DERMATOLOGISTS
4 Fitzroy Square
London W1T 5HQ
020 7383 0266
www.bad.org.uk
Provides a list of registered dermatologists; telephone callers only.

DIABETES UK
Macleod House
10 Parkway
London NW1 7AA
www.diabetes.org.uk
enquiries: 020 7424 1000:
careline: 0845 120 2960

FORESIGHT
Association for the Promotion of Preconceptual Care
178 Hawthorn Road
West Bognor
West Sussex PO21 2UY
01243 868001
www.foresight-preconception.org.uk
Advice on all aspects of preparing for pregnancy.

IBS (IRRITABLE BOWEL SYNDROME) NETWORK
Unit 5, 53 Mowbray Street
Sheffield S3 8EN
0114 272 3253: helpline
(Mon-Fri 6pm-8pm,
Sat 10-12 noon)
www.ibsnetwork.org.uk
An independent self-help group offering membership, advice, support and useful publications.

ME (MYALGIC ENCEPHALOMYELITIS) ASSOCIATION
4 Top Angel
Buckingham Industrial Park
Buckingham
Bucks MK18 1TH
0870 444 8233: info line
www.meassociation.org.uk
'Listening Ear' programme for people who need someone to talk to (afternoons, evenings and weekends).

NATIONAL ASSOCIATION FOR COLITIS AND CROHN'S DISEASE
4 Beaumont House
St Albans, Herts AL1 5HH
0845 130 2233
(Mon-Fri 10am-1pm)
www.nacc.org.uk
National charity supplying information and support.

NATIONAL ECZEMA SOCIETY
www.eczema.org.uk
email: info@eczema.org.uk
Online information and advice.

NATIONAL MULTIPLE SCLEROSIS SOCIETY
MS National Centre
372 Edgware Road
London NW2 6ND
020 8438 0700
helpline: 0808 800 8000
www.mssociety.org.uk
Information and support for people with MS and their families.

PARKINSON'S DISEASE SOCIETY
United Scientific House
215 Vauxhall Bridge Road
London SW1V 1EJ
020 7931 8080
0808 800 0303: helpline
www.parkinsons.org.uk
Support group and information service.

RAYNAUD'S AND SCLERODERMA ASSOCIATION
112 Crewe Road
Alsager
Cheshire ST7 2JA
01270 872776
www.raynauds.org.uk
Information pack, details of heating aids, research and treatment programme.

Suppliers of supplements and other products
HEALTH PLUS
Dolphin House
27 Cradle Hill Ind. Estate
Seaford
East Sussex BN25 3JE
01323 872277
www.healthplus.co.uk
Mail-order service.

HIGHER NATURE
Burwash Common
East Sussex TN19 7LX
01435 883484
www.highernature.co.uk
Supplies supplements and some books by mail order.

NATURE'S BEST
Century Place
Tunbridge Wells TN2 3BE
01892 552 118
nutrition advice: 01892 552175
www.naturesbest.co.uk
Vitamins and minerals by mail order.

THE NUTRI CENTRE
7 Park Crescent
London W1B 1PF
020 7436 5122
www.nutricentre.com
Supplies supplements, including DGL chewable liquorice tablets and homeopathic remedies.

Other useful organisations
THE SOIL ASSOCIATION
Bristol House
40-56 Victoria Street
Bristol BS1 6BY
0117 314 5000
www.soilassociation.org
Provides list of organic suppliers.

BREAKSPEAR HOSPITAL
Hertfordshire House
Wood Lane
Hemel Hempstead
Herts HP2 4FD
01442 261333
www.breakspearmedical.com
Private hospital offering treatment for allergies and environmentally induced conditions with emphasis on nutrition and supplements.

WEBSITES
It can be dangerous to follow medical advice given on the internet without first consulting your doctor. Sites run by established organisations are likely to be more reliable than those hosted by individuals. Many of the websites listed have searchable databases, links to other relevant sites and up-to-date information on specific ailments or nutritional and herbal medicine in general.

www.bmj.com
Current and archived issues of the *British Medical Journal* with searchable topics and links to related sites.

www.healthcentre.org.uk
Medical information site with some 4000 links to mostly UK sites covering a wide range of medical topics. Maintained by a GP in North Yorkshire.

www.healthfinder.gov
User-friendly US site with information on particular ailments and family health.

www.healthnotes.com
US complementary and integrative medicine site, with information on drug and nutrient interactions and details of research on herbal medicine and nutrition.

www.hebs.scot.nhs.uk
Information from the Health Education Board in Scotland, with a virtual health centre, searchable database of health information and advice about diet and drugs.

www.hsis.org
Health suppliers' information service for consumers and the media, with details of specific supplements, information about supplement myths and facts, and useful links. Coordinated by the Proprietary Association of Great Britain.

www.immunesupport.com
US site for sufferers from chronic fatigue syndrome and fibromyalgia; includes directory of support groups.

www.inciid.org
Site for the International Council on Infertility, based in the USA, offering fact sheets and a global directory of professionals in the field.

www.mca.gov.uk
A government site belonging to the Medicines and Health-care products Regulatory Agency (MHRA) dedicated to safety issues associated with herbal medicines. Gives general advice on the use of herbal remedies and also covers specific safety issues.

www.nhsdirect.nhs.uk
National Health Service site, covering the latest health stories and practical advice for healthy living and treating minor ailments at home, with a 24 hour nurse-led telephone advice service and online support.

www.nlm.nih.gov
US National Library of Medicine site, offering a searchable library of medical information with details of research programmes. Includes Medline (registration required), which has references from more than 4000 medical journals.

www.patient.co.uk
Site edited by two GPs which aims to give non-medically trained individuals information about health issues. Includes a section devoted to vitamins.

www.thinknatural.com
Comprehensive, searchable UK site with sections on vitamins, minerals and herbs, health features and an online shop.

Glossary

ABSORPTION The uptake by the body of a supplement, drug or other substance through the digestive tract, skin or mucous membranes.

ACUTE Short, severe, not chronic; designates an illness or condition typically lasting no more than a week or two.

AMINO ACIDS Chemical substances from which proteins are built. They are produced in the body and found in foods.

ANTIBIOTIC A drug that kills or inhibits infection-causing bacteria.

ANTICOAGULANT A drug, such as warfarin or aspirin, that deters blood clotting; often used by those at risk of heart attacks. Also known as a blood thinner.

ANTICONVULSANT A drug that prevents seizures; used to treat epilepsy.

ANTIFUNGAL A drug that combats athlete's foot or other infections caused by a fungus.

ANTI-INFLAMMATORY A drug or supplement that fights inflammation, a bodily response to injury or irritation, characterised by redness, heat, swelling and pain.

ANTIOXIDANT A substance that protects cells from the damaging effects of highly reactive molecules called free radicals. Some anti-oxidants are made by

the body; others, such as vitamins C and E, are obtained through diet or nutritional supplements.

ANTISEPTIC An infection-fighting herb, drug or other substance.

ANTISPASMODIC A drug or supplement that prevents spasms or cramps in the digestive tract or elsewhere.

ATHEROSCLEROSIS The build-up of cholesterol and other substances in the artery walls ('hardening of the arteries'), leading to heart disease, angina, heart attack, stroke and other ailments.

AUTOIMMUNE DISORDER An ailment, such as lupus or rheumatoid arthritis, in which the immune system mistakenly attacks the body's own healthy tissues.

BETA-BLOCKER A type of drug that affects the heart, blood vessels and other body parts; often prescribed to treat high blood pressure or angina.

BILE A fat-digesting substance produced in the liver, stored in the gall bladder, and released into the intestine when needed.

BOTANICAL A herb or plant with healing properties.

CAPILLARIES Tiny blood vessels that link veins and arteries. In the capillaries oxygen and nutrients are transferred from the blood to the cells, and waste products are removed.

CARTILAGE A dense yet flexible tissue in the joints, spine, throat, ears, nose and other areas. It is not as hard as bone, but it does provide protection and support.

CHOLESTEROL A fat-like substance that circulates in the blood and helps to build cell membranes; high levels can increase the risk of heart attack. *See also* HDL *and* LDL.

CHRONIC Persistent or long term; describes an illness or condition that often requires months or years of treatment.

COENZYME A substance that acts in concert with enzymes to speed up chemical reactions in the body.

COLLAGEN A tough, fibrous protein that provides support throughout the body and helps to form bones, cartilage, skin, joints and other tissues.

COMPLEX A combination of vitamins, minerals, herbs or other nutritional supplements. Examples include vitamin B complex, liver (lipotropic) complex and amino acid complex.

COMPRESS A soft cotton or flannel cloth or piece of gauze that has been soaked in a herbal tea or other healing substance, then folded and placed on the skin to help to reduce inflammation and pain.

DEMENTIA Loss of mental faculties as a result of Alzheimer's disease or other brain impairment.

DIURETIC A substance that draws water from the body tissues and increases the total output of urine.

DOUCHE A herbal tea, acidophilus and water mixture, for example, that can be used to flush the vagina; may be recommended for infections.

ENDORPHINS Natural pain-reducing substances released by the pituitary gland, producing an effect similar to that of narcotic pain relievers.

ENTERIC COATING A protective covering that enables a pill to pass intact through the stomach into the small intestine, where the coating dissolves and the contents are absorbed.

ENZYME A protein that speeds up specific chemical reactions and processes in the body, such as digestion and energy production.

ESSENTIAL FATTY ACIDS (EFAs) The building blocks that the body uses to make fats. To ensure good health the body must obtain various kinds of EFAs through diet or supplements (such as fish oils and flaxseed oil).

ESSENTIAL OIL A concentrated oil extracted from herbs or other plants.

EXPECTORANT A substance that makes it easier to cough up mucus.

EXTRACT A pill, powder, tincture or other form of a herb that contains a concentrated, and usually standard, amount of therapeutic ingredients.

FLAVONOIDS A large group of phytochemicals found in plants. Most are colourless, but some are pigments responsible for the colours of many fruits and vegetables.

FREE RADICALS Highly reactive and unstable molecules, generated in the body, that can damage cells, leading potentially to heart disease, cancer and other ailments. Antioxidants help to minimise the damage they cause.

GDU (GELATIN DIGESTING UNIT) A dosage measure for bromelain, a supplement that can help to reduce pain and inflammation. Potencies of bromelain are based on GDUs or MCUs (milk clotting units – *see below*). One GDU equals 1.5 MCU.

HAEMOGLOBIN The oxygen-carrying component of red blood cells. Made of iron and protein, it transports oxygen from the lungs to the cells.

HDL (HIGH DENSITY LIPOPROTEIN) One of two types of lipoprotein in the blood that transport cholesterol around the body. High levels of HDL – which carries much less fat than LDLs, or low density lipoproteins – signal a lower than average risk of heart disease. HDL cholesterol is also known as 'good' cholesterol. *See also* cholesterol *and* LDL.

HERB A plant or plant part – the leaves, stem, roots, bark, buds or flowers – which can be used for medicinal or other purposes (such as flavouring foods).

HOMOCYSTEINE An amino acid-like substance; high levels in the blood have been linked to heart disease.

HORMONE Any of various chemical messengers (produced by the ovaries, testes, adrenal, pituitary, thyroid and other glands) that have far-reaching effects throughout the body. Hormones regulate everything from growth and tissue repair to metabolism, reproduction and blood pressure, as well as the body's response to stress.

HORMONE REPLACEMENT THERAPY (HRT) The use of supplemental oestrogen and progesterone (in the form of progestogen) – female sex hormones – to relieve the adverse effects of the menopause. The therapy may also help to prevent osteoporosis.

IMMUNE RESPONSE The body's natural defence system against infectious microbes – including disease-causing bacteria and viruses – as well as cancer cells within the body itself.

INSULIN RESISTANCE A condition in which the body's cells do not respond adequately to the hormone insulin. It can lead to higher blood sugar (glucose) levels, increased insulin production by the pancreas and, possibly, diabetes.

INTERFERONS Virus-fighting proteins that are produced by the immune system.

INTERNATIONAL UNIT (IU) A dose of a vitamin that produces a standard physiological response, irrespective of the chemical form that is administered (Most commonly used for vitamin E, which has several different chemical forms.)

JAUNDICE A symptom of hepatitis and other liver disorders, marked by a yellow hue to the skin and eyes.

LDL (LOW DENSITY LIPOPROTEIN) One of two types of lipoprotein in the blood that transport cholesterol around the body. LDLs carry about three-quarters of the cholesterol in the blood. High LDL levels usually reflect high cholesterol levels and imply a higher risk of heart disease. LDL cholesterol is also known as 'bad' cholesterol. *See also* cholesterol *and* HDL.

LIPOTROPIC COMBINATION A 'fat-digesting' blend of choline, inositol, methionine, milk thistle and other nutrients used to promote the health of the liver. Also called liver complex.

MACROPHAGE A type of white blood cell that can surround and digest disease-causing bacteria and other foreign microbes.

MCU (MILK CLOTTING UNIT) A dosage measure for bromelain, a supplement that can help to reduce pain and inflammation. *See also* GDU.

METABOLISM The sum of all the chemical changes that occur within the living body. (There are two directions: anabolism is the formation of more complex molecules; catabolism is the formation of less complex molecules.)

MICROGRAM (MCG) A metric measure of weight used in dosages; sometimes denoted by the symbol μ. There are 1000 mcg in 1 milligram (mg).

MINERAL An inorganic substance, such as calcium, found in the earth's crust that plays a crucial role in the human body for enzyme creation, regulation of heart rhythm, bone formation, digestion and other meta-bolic processes.

MIXED AMINO ACIDS A balanced blend (complex) of amino acids, often taken in conjunction with individual amino acid supplements.

MONOAMINE-OXIDASE (MAO) INHIBITOR A specific class of drug used to treat depression, frequently interacting with foods, drugs and supplements.

MUCOUS MEMBRANES The pink, moist, skinlike layers that line the lips, mouth, vagina, eyelids and other body cavities and passages.

NEURALGIA Sharp, some-times severe pain resulting from damage to a nerve and often affecting a specific area of the body, such as the face.

NEUROTRANSMITTER Any of various chemicals found in the brain and throughout the body that transmit signals among nerve cells.

NONSTEROIDAL ANTI-INFLAMMATORY DRUG (NSAID) A drug such as aspirin or ibuprofen that reduces inflammation and pain by blocking the pro-duction of prostaglandins. *See also* prostaglandins.

NUTRITIONAL SUPPLEMENT A nutrient that has been synthesised in the laboratory or extracted from plants or animals for medicinal use.

OESTROGEN A female sex hormone, produced mainly in the ovaries, that helps to regulate menstruation, reproduction and other processes.

OLIGOMERIC PROANTHO-CYANIDIN COMPLEXES (OPCS) A group of anti-oxidant compounds, also called proanthocyanidins – found in pine bark, grape seed extract, green tea, red wine and other substances – that may help to protect against heart and vascular disease.

OVER-THE-COUNTER (OTC) A drug that can be sold without a doctor's prescription.

PHYTOCHEMICALS Substances found in fruits, vegetables, grains, herbs and other plants that may help to protect against cancer, heart disease and other ailments.

PHYTOESTROGENS Compounds present in soya and other plants that have mild oestrogenic properties. They can help to alleviate the symptoms of hormonal imbalance in women, and may reduce the risk of certain cancers.

PLACEBO A substance that contains no medicinal ingredients. Often used in scientific studies as a control so that the effects of the drug or supplement under study can be compared with the untreated body.

POULTICE A soft, moist substance spread between layers of cloth or gauze and applied, usually heated, to the skin. Poultices can be used to reduce pain and inflammation, to treat bruises and to promote the healing of wounds and the extraction of pus.

PROBIOTICS Cultures of 'friendly' bacteria normally found in the intestine. Pro-biotics such as acidophilus and bifidus are consumed to improve digestion by multiplying and restoring the balance of the normal bacterial population of the intestine.

PROGESTERONE A female sex hormone, made by the ovaries, that helps to regulate menstruation. Progesterone belongs to the group of hormones known as progestogens, which are syn-thesised for therapeutic use.

PROLACTIN A hormone secreted by the pituitary gland whose level is raised by stress; prolactin is also involved in promoting lactation.

PROSTAGLANDINS Hormone-like chemicals produced naturally in the body in response to a stimulus. Their wide range of effects include inducing inflammation, stimulating uterine contractions during labour and protecting the lining of the stomach.

RECOMMENDED DAILY ALLOWANCE (RDA) An average of a key nutrient that people should obtain from their diets, established according to European Union regulations. RDAs apply to 'average adults' and take no account of individual nutritional requirements. They are used on labels only; Reference Nutrient Intakes (RNIs) are used for all other purposes.

REFERENCE NUTRIENT INTAKE (RNI) The daily amount of a vitamin or mineral needed by healthy individuals to meet the body's requirements and prevent a deficiency. These guidelines are set by the Department of Health.

STANDARDISED EXTRACT A concentrated form of a herb that contains a set (standardised) level of active ingredients. Standardisation helps to guarantee a consistent dosage strength, or potency, from one batch of herb to the next. Standardised extracts are available only for certain herbs, either as pills or tinctures, or in other forms.

STEROIDS A common name for corticosteroids, inflammation-fighting drugs that are sometimes prescribed to treat allergic reactions, asthma, skin rashes, multiple sclerosis, lupus and other ailments.

SUBLINGUAL Beneath the tongue. Some supplements, such as vitamin B_{12}, are formulated to dissolve in the mouth, allowing swift absorption into the blood-stream. This means that the supplement avoids metabo-lism in the liver, which can reduce circulating levels.

TANNIN An astringent substance derived from plants that can contract blood vessels and body tissues.

TESTOSTERONE The principal male sex hormone, produced in the testes, that induces changes at puberty and helps to build strong muscles and bones. Women also make a small amount of testosterone in their ovaries.

THERAPEUTIC DOSE The amount of a vitamin, mineral, herb, nutritional supplement or drug needed to produce a desired healing effect (as opposed to the minimum amount needed to prevent a deficiency – such as the RNI, for example).

TINCTURE A liquid usually made by soaking a whole herb or its parts in a mixture of water and ethyl alcohol (such as vodka). The alcohol helps to extract the herb's active components, concen-trating and preserving them.

TONIC A herb (such as ginseng) or herbal blend that is used to 'tone' the body or a specific organ, imparting added strength or vitality.

TRICLYCERIDE The chemical term for fat. People who have high triclyceride levels in their blood increase the likelihood of developing heart disease.

VITAMIN An organic substance that plays an essential role in regulating cell functions throughout the body. Most vitamins must be ingested in food or supplements because the body cannot produce them.

Index

Acknowledgments

Healing Supplements is based on *Reader's Digest Guide to Vitamins, Minerals and Supplements*, published by The Reader's Digest Association Limited, London

First edition Copyright © 2006

The Reader's Digest Association Limited,
11 Westferry Circus, Canary Wharf, London E14 4HE
www.readersdigest.co.uk

We are committed to both the quality of our products and the service we provide to our customers.
We value your comments, so please feel free to contact us on 08705 113366 or via our website at www.readersdigest.co.uk
If you have any comments about the content of our books, you can contact us at gbeditorial@readersdigest.co.uk

NOTE TO READERS

While the creators of this work have made every effort to be as accurate and up to date as possible, medical and pharmacological knowledge is constantly changing. Readers are recommended to consult a qualified medical specialist for individual advice. The writers, researchers, editors and the publishers of this work cannot be held liable for any errors and omissions, or actions that may be taken as a consequence of information contained within this work.

CHIEF CONSULTANTS:
Dr Alan Lakin MSc PhD CChem FRSC FRSH MIFST
Dr Ann Walker MSc PhD MIFST FRSH CBiol MIBiol
  MNIMH MCPP
Dr John Cormack BDS MB BS MRCS LRCP

PROJECT EDITOR Rachel Warren Chadd
ART EDITOR Louise Turpin
INDEXER Hilary Bird
PROOFREADER Barry Gage

READER'S DIGEST GENERAL BOOKS, LONDON
EDITORIAL DIRECTOR Julian Browne
ART DIRECTOR Nick Clark
MANAGING EDITOR Alastair Holmes
HEAD OF BOOK DEVELOPMENT Sarah Bloxham
PICTURE RESOURCE MANAGER Sarah Stewart-Richardson
PRE-PRESS ACCOUNT MANAGER Sandra Fuller
PRODUCT PRODUCTION MANAGER Claudette Bramble
SENIOR PRODUCTION CONTROLLER Deborah Trott

ORIGINATION Colour Systems Ltd, London
PRINTING AND BINDING Arvato Iberia, Europe

PICTURE CREDITS

The publishers would like to thank the following for providing the illustrations in Vitamins, Minerals and Supplements. All images are Reader's Digest © except for those from GettyOne Photodisc

Martin Norris: 11BC, 12B, 14, 15, 16, 19, 32, 41, 44, 52, 53, 55, 56, 60, 64, 73, 86TL, 86BL, 87, 90, 96, 110, 130, 134TL, 138, 144 (pills), 146, 152, 156, 160, 162, 174, 175

Digital Vision front cover, 6

GettyOne Photodisc: 7, 8, 11, 21, 30, 134, 135, 136, 137

All other photographs are by Lisa Koenig

Book Code 400-308-01
ISBN-10 0 276 44185 0
ISBN-13 978 0 276 44185 1
Oracle Code 250009956S.00.24